Angel Guidance ~ Messages of Love and Healing

Published in the United States by BookLocker.com, Inc., Port Charlotte, Florida.

The author and publisher of this book do not dispense medical advice or prescribe any technique as a form of treatment for physical or emotional problems and therefore assume no responsibility for your actions. The intent of this material is to provide general information to help your mental, emotional and spiritual growth. WE encourage you to seek professional assistance for all areas of healing.

Editing: Angela Williams and Sharon Taphorn

Cover design: Todd Engel

Printed in the United States of America on acid-free paper.

Shifting Times Media 2012

www.playingwiththeuniverse.com

First Edition

Angel Guidance ~ Messages of Love and Healing

Sharon Taphorn

Introduction

I had never really planned to work as an ambassador for the angelic realm. I've always been aware of the guides and angels; however felt I was supposed to work more with the guidance realm. My mother had gifted me with a few decks of Angel Cards from Doreen Virtue a few years back that I really didn't use that much. Mainly they sat on my coffee table for friends and clients to choose one or two for themselves when they came over for a reading or a class. Then one day I was doing a special for a radio station I was broadcasting one of my shows on and we needed time fillers between guests. I pulled a card from one of the decks for the listener's in between interviews. They were very well received and helpful. They were such a hit I decided to add them to one of my shows at the end. A few weeks later while I was blogging on a spiritual community I was feeling a bit sad that everything on the site seemed to be about self promotion and not really helping the readers. So, the angels said, 'Why don't you put up a message that has no other agenda other than helping people?" That was the beginning of the Angel Card of the Day. A few months after posting a card, I began to feel that the messages should be more than just sharing someone else's work and I began to write the messages that the angels gave me instead of what the cards said. So, I changed the name to Angel Wisdom of the Day to reflect the evolution. I had not intended to add my name to them until someone else named Sharon decided to do a card each day and I didn't want any confusion about our work. I was also gathering a larger audience and was finding my work on many sites. So the angels suggested I add my name since I was doing so much work with them.

Also shortly after, the angels asked me to start a radio program based on the wisdom and other spiritual information. So, being the adventurous warrior that I am, I began the program "Calling All Angels", and the angels would help me to host a program that was more like a workshop on working with angels, getting to know the angels, assignments from the Angels, meditations and readings. And now, they guided me to produce this book.

And thus began my journey with working with the angels. I am honoured to share their wisdom, and how to work with them with my readers and listeners. It has helped countless people find their voice, clarity and passion, as well as me to find mine. I was once asked how I knew the messages come from the angels, and my response was, "When I get the messages I am surrounded by this love that is nothing like I've ever experienced on the earth plane and that is how I can tell the difference."

I want to also thank Diana Cooper and Doreen Virtue for all the beauty and the wisdom they have shared through their books and cards as are an endless resource for me.

Please enjoy the wisdom, love, empowerment and healing that is embedded upon these pages.

Love and blessings, Sharon and the angels

This book can be read from front to back, used as a reference guide, or daily inspiration. You can start with day one or simply pick up the book, flip through the pages and let the angels guide you to what spirit wants you to know. Meditate on the message and invite the angels into each new day.

To my dad, Don Taphorn

My angel in heaven...I miss you everyday

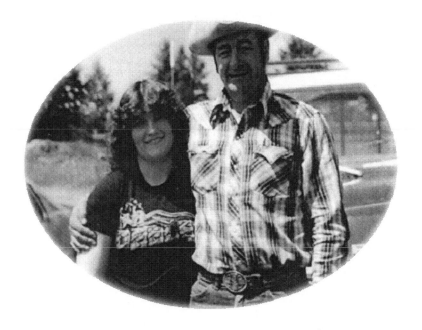

I know that you are always with me in my heart and guiding me.

I love you forever

With Thanks and Appreciation

I would like to acknowledge, first and foremost the angels and guides for your prodding and guiding me in the direction of my dreams and allowing me to be a conduit of your messages.

Thank you to all my loyal readers of the daily Angel Wisdom. Your questions and comments have allowed me to grow and expand my light as well as becoming a clearer channel.

Thank you to all the listeners and supporters of 'Calling All Angels'. It is for you that we do this work. We are so honoured to assist you in awakening and evolving. Your love and support make all things possible in my world as well.

Thank you to my mother, Carol Taphorn, for so many things. Thank you for agreeing to be my mother and supporting me throughout my life. Thank you for your love, wisdom and understanding. Thank you for the guidance and for teaching me to discern and not shut down my abilities to communicate with other realms.

Thank you to my sister, Angela Williams for your love and support and all the time you spend reading and editing my books and articles. I so admire your strength and tenacity. Thank you for being my sister and my friend.

To my son Nicholas Taphorn, my greatest teacher, without you being exactly who you are, I would not be who I am. It is because of you that I am possible. Thank you for being my son. I love you forever.

Thank you to the human angels who have deeply affected my life, been a support and true human angel to me. Without you in my life, I think I might have abandoned the earth mission and returned home. Thank you for your friendship and support as this beautiful journey unfolds. In no particular order, I am honoured to call you family and friend: To all of my family, thank you, Kari McCuish, Beverly Cohoon, Steve and Barbara Rother, Debbie VanSummeren-Morgan, Kim Callander Giesbrecht, Brandon Miller, Kendall Farrell, Angele Ortega of Issues Magazine, Maria Carr of Ok In Health Magazine, Qiming Wuu, Kahu Fred Sterling, Dr. Eve Kacamarek, Karen Maher, Sue Peters, Donna Rode, Cyndi Jacob, Denise St. Laurent, Lourisha Shaw.

And, thank you Robert, Missy, Alissa and Jessie Galloway-Taphorn for getting up for 8am every Saturday morning during summer break to help me with my booth.

Thank you to my spiritual family. From my heart, I am deeply grateful for the love and support of all the people, both named and unnamed, who have worked with me to share the messages of the angels and to let others know that they are never alone, dearly loved and always supported. We are all a part of each other and together in this quest call Life.

Many of these messages were written during my healing journey and helped me through many dark nights of pain. Thank you to the angels for helping me to heal.

1

Happy New Year

Each of you is raising your personal vibrations. Each new cycle is like starting a new year. As you do, you are becoming more sensitive to your environment, new psychic and spiritual experiences are changing the way you view life, the Universe and everything. Allow your spiritual gifts to open through study, prayer, and most importantly, meditation.

Remember you are a powerful, loving, and creative child of the Creator, all of you, in every weave, in every way and that you are loved far more than you could ever imagine. This year is an opportunity to expand your light at an ever increasing pace. Embrace the opportunities that we together put before you.

Affirmation: "I am powerful. I am having new psychic and spiritual experiences."

2

We are with you

Ask your Angels for assistance. We are always here and we are always ready to help. However, we must be asked in order to assist. We must always be invited into the human realm in order to help you. We are with you now, giving you the courage to make life changes that will help you work on your Divine life purpose. Be open to receiving Divine guidance and assistance. You deserve it.

Use the power of your imagination to help you visualize and connect with us. Use your heart energy to connect with us and trust the images and/or feelings that you receive, they are trustworthy, and you are worthy.

Affirmation: "I am surrounded by angelic support and I quickly notice the signs they offer my. I am worthy to receive."

3

Meditation

Spend time alone in nature if you can. Meditate upon your desires and intentions. Meditation is our way of communicating with you; assisting you and helping you see the bigger picture. Ask the angels to help you gain a positive perspective. Create affirmations to assist you in reaching those desires.

Welcome the feelings of peace. Allow for a new tranquility and a smoother road ahead as you continue to practice and breath daily. Use the power of your chosen affirmations and do a small act each day that leads your closer to your desired outcome.

Affirmation: "I receive wonderful guidance and healing during my meditations."

4

Time to let go

The sun sets and rises each day. As it is the same with the adventures in your life. See the beauty and the gifts within each moment; know that the sun will rise again tomorrow, and then the next day, and the day after that. Endings are merely the start of a new beginning, and your angels surround you every step of the way. You are never alone and always supported. Let go of those things that don't serve who you are becoming or that hold you back from receiving the results you desire.

As you experience enormous change through releasing, it is important to cleanse and detoxify any part of your life, the physical world, where your thoughts are and what is your spiritual practice. Know that your desired outcomes are achieved as you keep up the good work of releasing and letting go.

Affirmation: "I forgive myself, knowing that I did the best I knew how at the time and I am ready for wonderful new experiences as I move forward."

5

Take action

Trust in your truth. Trust your feelings and your gut instincts and lovingly assert yourself. We will guide you through the actions that are necessary. Your focus is to avoid procrastination at all costs. Break things down into baby steps so that you do not become overwhelmed. Then, each day take those steps, for every step makes a difference.

You already know what to do, and you have made up your mind to take action. We are here to validate that your decisions are on the path of Light and to support you along the way. Sometimes you may feel too emotional or tired to take action. This is because you are unsure of the 'correct' way to go or feel uncertain about what you want. These are the moments to call upon us to strengthen you. We are always by your side waiting to give you strength and courage and love.

Affirmation: "I have the faith to live my truth; I am willing to do those things that bring me joy."

6

Inner wisdom

Angel guidance reminds you that everyone can connect to their inner wisdom. Ask us to illuminate you and help you to connect with your own deep knowing. Connect with the golden ray of wisdom drawing from source energy. Visualize yourself surrounded in a cloak of golden light, take some slow, deep breaths, feel your inner core strengthen and shine and tap into the wisdom that is available to you there. Let the light wash away any negativity and you will become more open minded, clear and wise.

Wear your golden cloak of wisdom any time you wish to study any kind of wisdom or class, as this will assist you in absorbing the information faster and easier. Divine assistance is available to you now. Ask, and you shall receive.

Affirmation: "I am connected to my inner wisdom at all times. I only need to quiet myself for a second and the connection is immediately available to me."

7

Choose peace

We are the angels of Peace. We bring to you new tranquility; and a smoother road ahead. Oftentimes after a period of a lot of energy and sometimes turmoil you can become tired. Your mind and body crave peace and quiet, and we angels are here to help you with that desire. We can give you new opportunities to spend time alone, meditating upon what you truly desire, and relax your mind and body, and open your heart. We will bring you peace and tranquility to your heart and soul so that you can mirror the peace of mind that is your true Divine self.

This inner foundation of peace has a powerful healing affect. Give any cares or worries to your angels and allow us to take your stress and burdens. Your outer life will begin to reflect your inner peacefulness. Smooth roads are ahead for you, and the worst is now behind you. A new day is dawning each day, a fresh new start with a peaceful perspective.

Affirmation: "Shanti, Shanti, Shanti. I choose to be tranquil and I am a peaceful person."

(Shanti is Sanskrit and means peace, rest, calmness, tranquility, or bliss. Source Wikipedia)

8

Follow your dreams

We are leading you toward the answers to your prayers. Please listen to and follow the promptings you feel or hear, as we are communicating to you though your intuition, thoughts, dreams, and meditations. Take time out to relax and get really clear on your desires and dreams so that we are guiding you with clear pictures of your desires. You are surrounded by help on so many levels. Look around and think of who in your circles is best able and willing to help you with your venture, and initiate contact.

Notice any repetitious thoughts and feelings, or vivid visions, dreams or auditory messages that you hear in your head or from others or even in songs. These are our loving messages, urging you to take action or make changes. We will make sure that you are safe while you follow your Divine guidance.

See yourself and others through the eyes of the angels, in unconditional love and acceptance.

Affirmation: "I Trust the vision of my potential and of myself expanding each day."

9

Trust

Your prayers are manifesting. Remain positive and follow your guidance. Your guidance is trustworthy. Perhaps you have received a wonderful idea as an answer to your prayers, or you are working on a new romance with a spiritual basis or enhancing your current relationship.

This guidance is trustworthy. Now is the time to act on this fertile energy. The angels are here to assist you every step of the way. Ask for and be open to receiving our support for anything that you need related to these projects. This is a precious time for you and your dreams. You don't have to strain or push to make them come true. Trust that it is yours.

Angel wisdom reminds you that you have an entourage of energies wishing to be a part of your journey. Your guardian angels want you to know how much they love you. Your angels love is completely unconditional and all encompassing. They never judge or abandon you. The angels are simply here to support you so that you can spiritually grow.

Affirmation: "I receive trustworthy guidance; I feel the love from my entourage of angels."

10

Healing and releasing

Your emotions are healing and this process almost feels like your heart physically hurts. This is opening you up your heart chakra to greater love. Ask your angels to help you release any anger and unforgiveness from your heart and also your mind. Having thoughts of unforgiveness for yourself and others creates toxic energy that will live within your very cells until it is released and transformed.

Angel guidance reminds you that your soul desires only to joyfully serve and to swim in a constant stream of joy and love. This stream continuously feeds you everything you need. So, put your entire focus on getting to and staying in this stream of balanced giving and receiving. Be gentle with yourself as you get there, for this is not a race or competition, everyone wins.

Trust is one of the highest forces in the Universe, along with joy. During this period of healing, release, relax and take stock of where you've been and where it is that you wish to go. This will give you a chance to reflect on the way ahead, strengthen yourself and prepare for the next stage of your journey.

Affirmation: "I forgive myself. I Release that which no longer serves who I am becoming."

11

Curiosity

See life through the curious eyes of a child.

Seeing life through a child lets you see the excitement and wonder that is always around you. Curiosity keeps you alive, interested and interesting.

The angels invite you to be curious about yourself as this allows you to explore who you are and where you are going. Be interested in the people that surround you.

The Universe is a continuous source of fascination. Be curious about the wonderful Universe in which you live. Be curious about your angels and their Divine role in your plans. See the beauty that is all around you, always.

The radiant delight of a child, the first time they discover or experience something new is breathtaking, so spend time today experiencing everything as if it is the first time you seen the world from this vantage point and the radiance of your delight will illuminate you.

Affirmation: "I explore the wonder and beauty that is all around me."

12

Be persistent

What do you desire right now? Visualize it, and it will come your way. Angel wisdom reminds you that negativity will block your progress. If you have been asking your angels, 'What is next for me?' we wish to also remind you that we are waiting for you to make that decision for yourself. If you have been feeling stuck lately, it is probably because you have not decided where to go next. We can show you options, however the choice is ultimately up to you. An impasse can occur if you are afraid to make the wrong choice. There is no wrong choice; there are just choices that take longer than others, however these are often the paths that teach you the most. We will light the path of your choosing. Your mission is to choose the path **you** wish to take.

If you are not sure what is the next best step to take, take a time out to play, sing or laugh, for all of these activities will give you the retreat from your activities and allow us the opportunity to infuse your creativity.

And once you have decided what to do next, we will assist you through your intuition, signs and inspirations as you take the steps that lead you closer to your desires. Stay positive and visualize your dreams as if they are already manifested and keep on going. You can do it. Commit to making your dreams your experience.

Affirmation: "Everything I do brings me closer to my dreams and desires."

13

Giving and receiving

Are you're giving and receiving in balance?

Angel wisdom reminds you that keeping you're giving and receiving in balance can sometimes be a challenge; however it is so important for your peace and wellbeing. The entire Universe works on cycles of balance, similar to your inhalations and exhalations. When you only exhale (give) or inhale (receive), you become out of rhythm with the Universe.

For optimal health, energy, vitality and peace of mind, it is important to keep your giving and receiving ratio in balance. Most Lightworkers have a challenge in receiving more than giving. If you find this out of balance, take a deep breath and know that is okay to receive. Say "thank you" graciously even if it feels uncomfortable at first. Remember, you don't have to do this journey by yourself. We are here to assist you; as well there are human angels who are all around you waiting to help.

If you are receiving more than you are giving, find a worthwhile charity, or consciously choose to give to others each day to bring this back into balance. It is so wonderful to receive and that is part of the universal balance. It is also important to give something of yourself to others too. Ask yourself and your angels, "How may I serve?", and swim in the constant stream of bliss that giving and receiving provide.

Celebrate each breath, and say thank you.

Affirmation: "I now give and receive graciously."

14

Trust

Your desired outcome will occur. Have patience and trust; don't try to force things to happen. Detach from your desires once you have made your decisions and trust that your angels will take care of the details. Your responsibility is to: ask for help from your guides and angels, and you all have an entourage of light beings in various forms and from various dimensions who have agreed to be your assistance from the other side.

The second is pay attention to your inner guidance. Connect with your own deep knowing and you will be guided each step of the way. We talk to you through the prompting of spirit and your inner guidance is connected to us. So wear your golden cloak of wisdom always.

Be sure that you are not blocking your manifestations with contradictory negative thoughts. Use positive affirmations to help you stay focused, positive and strong. Sometimes situations that appear negative to you are your opportunities to grow and expand your ability to be more love. So remember to see only the love within it, be brave and look at what your next step is with us by your side.

Affirmation: "I trust in the support of the Universe."

15

Change

It is time to release the past. Let go of anything that no longer serve the new you that is now emerging. These current changes involve making swift decisions and taking action now, and will let the new you begin to thrive in the place of your old self. Any actions and people from the past you are being urged to let go of now. Soon enough the purpose of this process, difficult as it may seem, will become clear and you will understand that in order to grow and bloom anew, this process and the energy that it creates is destined to work magic in your evolution.

You can do it. Release any doubts, it will help you realize your full potential, it is good to be taken out of your comfort zone, it won't last forever and resistance to change only brings more confusion in the energy around you, and when you make the necessary changes, watch what you will achieve when you finally give in to the process.

Now is the time for you to shine, and this process of change will help to create energy and strength for new projects, new loves, new friends and a new life purpose. Begin your new year by releasing the old so that all that you desire to create has room to grow.

Affirmation: "I release all doubts and disappointments. I deserve to have a wonderful life of abundance, good friends, meaningful activities that feed my soul, and I do."

16

Take a time out and enjoy

Take a time out and enjoy the results of the hard work you've been doing lately, or to rethink and plan what you are going to be doing next.

If you stop, slow down, or change direction, it doesn't mean you're in any way defeated or that you failed, in fact, it is a kind of triumph. You are worth it. Take good care of your health, and while there is definitely meaning in work well done, you are searching for something more spiritual right now. Start reading articles and books to help you grow, take time out for yourself, take a class that will expand your connection with yourself and turn your face to the sun. Take a walk in the woods. Enjoy your loved ones, your food, and care for your health.

Angel wisdom reminds you Life is complex, and yet so simple. Take the time to seek guidance and wise counsel, tune into your intuition and see what it is telling you about the path that you are currently on. Go on a spirit quest, you are worth it. Then, tap into the new stream of growth that is beginning for you.

Affirmation: "I have time and energy for myself to grow and expand my light."

17

Forgiveness

Sometimes we encounter challenging people and situations.

Angel guidance reminds you that these situations are often sent to you as a result of your prayers and desire to grow. These people are often your greatest teachers and part of your soul family. Your soul families are beings who love you the most and are willing to come to earth and be a part of your journey. Without your soul family assisting you, your soul would not grow.

Your guidance is to let go of the hurt, resentment and any anger from the past or present. When you forgive others and yourself, you enjoy love in your heart and lightness in your spirit.

You are safe and protected, always, regardless of how things appear. Ask your angels to assist you if your confidence and trust waivers.

When you love unconditionally, there is nothing to forgive. Love is for giving, so open your heart and give your love. Ask your angels to help you see people and events through their eyes and they will assist you. Forgiveness doesn't mean that what someone did to you is okay, it means that you are no longer willing to carry this burden in your heart and you want to heal.

Affirmation: "I forgive and love myself; I forgive and love you and all things unconditionally. I am free."

18

Family

Family includes your soul family. Our families are our greatest teachers, for these are the ones who love us the most. If you are experiencing any dramas or difficulties within your family, we can assist you in understanding and healing. Your angels wish to remind you that these are the experiences that have the greatest influence on your soul growth and that they are contracts made eons ago. These are the beings of light who love you the most, even if you are not aware who they truly are while not in physicality.

It is time to emerge beyond what can be seen by the physical or mental body. See them with your emotional and spiritual bodies.

In your mind and your heart, surround yourself, the people involved and the experience with calming light and many angels. Be open to the gifts within the situations, and allow yourself to feel peace and calmness once again. You can't choose how others react, only how you choose to respond.

You are dearly loved and never alone, so invoke our presence anytime you feel you need support, courage, and love.

Affirmation: "My family supports my soul's growth."

19

You are deserving of all your desires.

You deserve the best. Reach for the starts with your dreams and desires. As you reach for your dreams, believe that you are indeed deserving of these goals and they can't help but come true. Focus your intent and energy towards your creations and don't compromise your beliefs and desires. Trust that you deserve everything this beautiful Universe has to offer.

Your angel guidance is to find a quiet space for contemplation and look within for your hearts true desires. Reflect on the way ahead, strengthen yourself and prepare for the next phase of your life. Become aware of your gifts, your inner beauty and your wisdom. It is time for healing and creating your desires.

Affirmation: "I am deserving of all that I choose to create. I am worthy. I am capable. I AM."

20

Clear Intentions

Stay focused upon your intentions, desires, and priorities. Pay attention to the doors that are opening, and learn from the doors that are closing. Keep a positive outlook about your dreams, and imagine that they've already manifested into reality. Spend time each day devoted to projects that are dear to your heart.

If you are stuck or indecisive, the Universe doesn't know what you want. It is important to clearly decide what direction or goals you choose and then focus on them, creating an energy that is stronger.

If you are unsure what the next step on your path is, ask your angels. We will help to guide you. It is your responsibility to take the steps through those doors you choose take. Know that everything works within the Universal Laws, such as the Law of Attraction and the Law of Divine Timing. This means that the vibration you are putting out is what you receive, and that certain pieces of the puzzle must be in place so that other parts can come into play. If you skip, rush or ignore certain pieces or parts, the plan lacks a solid foundation, and you don't see the results you desire.

Decisiveness is the catalyst for the angels to clear the way for your manifestations. Let go of any fears or the worries and focus only on the destination you intend to reach. Enjoy the journey along the way.

Affirmation: "I project into the Universe that which I desire mirrored back to me."

21

Balance

Are you tired of juggling? Or, riding the proverbial roller coaster of emotions, thoughts or finances, or perhaps all three?

Look for the resolutions that are available to you now. Angel wisdom reminds you to bring balance, harmony and temperance into all aspects of your life.

Your angel guidance is to remember that life's journey can be what you make it. If you see only negative things, you will feel that you have bleak prospects in your future. If you feel the world is cruel and punishing, you will encounter lots of opportunities to see misfortune and anger, if you feel love and joy; you will see people who are happy, successful and expanding.

There is plenty of energy around that assists in seeing what you are feeling or resonating it back to you. Where are your thoughts? What is the world mirroring back to you? Do you see love?

Angel guidance says that now is the time to work on making life changes in how you see the world. Focus on being more conscious about where your thoughts are and where you want them to be. Be open to new ways and ideas from others who emulate those ideals and walk the talk in life.

The quest for balance and harmony can be challenging. It requires a certain kind of calm, steady approach and an almost scientific formula to understand the components that will help you plan a way to balance and harmonize your life. If you think creatively, and then use a well thought out plan, you can bring seemingly opposing elements into harmony, whether its friends and family, aspects of your own personality, or your work life. There is a way to transform your life: if you can fuse creativity and organization, you'll create a wealth of opportunity and enjoyment in your life. This is the year to find that perfect balance in your journey.

Affirmation: "I have enough discipline in my life to create the balance and harmony that I desire."

22

Honour yourself

Honour yourself and follow your guidance. Many of you have been undergoing tremendous spiritual growth. With all the shifts and changes that have been happening to you, you will begin to honour yourself more and trust your inner guidance. The more you use and trust your inner wisdom, the more it grows. Whatever you feed shall grow exponentially, and we see so much happening on your earth plane by those of you who are becoming so bright.

Take some time today to go out and play. Being out of doors and having some fun will assist in your shifts. You are able to breathe fresh air and expand your lungs as you run about laughing and enjoying yourself and from this, fresh new ideas pop into your head from your entourage of Light Beings, as well as your higher self. Drink plenty of life giving water too.

As you find more joy on journey each day becomes brighter than the one before it.

Affirmation: "I connect and trust my inner wisdom. I am vibrating at higher levels each day. I honour and love myself."

23

Light

Light illuminates darkness and gloom, bringing hope and inspiration. One candle can light an entire room of darkness, just as the lighthouse guides the ships to safety, your light can help to guide others along the way and also lighten your experience too.

Ask the angels to fill you with more light, for it contains spiritual information and knowledge. These are keys to the Universe and bring love and peace, as well as unlocking the wisdom within you. As your light becomes stronger and clearer, you will find clarity and purpose.

You will radiate brightly and become a beacon, reminding others of the Divine help that is available to all.

Angel wisdom suggests you ask the angels to ignite and strengthen the Divine flame that burns within you.

Affirmation: "Each day I expand my light with love. My light shines brightly to help others along the way."

24

Focused intent

Your desires are like paintings on the canvas of life. Take some time to meditate and pray, and contemplate what is next. If you are unsure of what is the next best step for you to take, consult an expert who can assist you in seeing the bigger picture that is before you. Your angels can assist with this endeavour, however if you are not sure or completely trust what you receive, then find a human angel who can assist you.

Do not be afraid of making the wrong decision, for there is never truly a wrong step to take. Angel wisdom reminds you that making no decision is the same as saying to the Universe that you want for everything to stay the same, and that is the energy that you will attract. Few things are as powerful as focused intent, visualize it, and feel it and it will come.

Seek the Divine within every situation as this cultivates the quality of joy and you become aware of the wonder of creation. Delight in everything. Enjoy the process of creation and enjoy life.

Affirmation: "I see the joy in every step of creating that which I desire. I am always free to choose again."

25

Golden opportunities

Important doors are opening for you now. Go forward and walk through them now as these are the answers to your prayers. You have been praying to your angels and asking for guidance on which is the next best step for you to take and we say that it is in front of you. Your mission is to now pay attention to the signs. These signs can come in the form of hunches, repetitious messages, words you hear in a song, words from another person or things you read. Pay attention to anything drawn to 3 or more times (sometimes you don't trust in the message so we have to give it to you in many different ways until you realize it is there).

We ask that you open your heart to love and use this as the mechanism you use to filter through the ideas and inspirations you feel. Close your eyes and allow us to open up this area to receive the higher energies and feel our love and admiration for you who does the earth journey. Then, carry that love with you throughout your day.

If you feel taxed or overwhelmed, take a moment and open your heart and feel our love once again, and then share that love with those around you. Not in a loud way, but with a gentle smile and beam it all around you. Share your golden self as you create. See the beauty within those moments.

Affirmation: "I see love and beauty all around me. I am surrounded by loving light as I move forward and walk

through the doors of the opportunities that open before me."

26

Happy endings

Change happens, whether you are ready or not. Focus on the happy endings at the end of each rainbow, for if it did not rain, you would not be gifted with beautiful flowers and trees, and grass, and waterfalls, and rainbows. You get the picture. The sun will rise again tomorrow. Angel wisdom reminds you to look for the beauty around you and keep your thoughts on those things that bring you joy.

Value yourself, expect success, or at the very least a conclusion that results in balance. Remember that you are a wonderful child of the Creator, you are likeable and loveable. Radiate a golden aura around you and know that the changes you are going through offer you an opportunity to grow. Stand tall and be confident. Ask your angels to step into your aura and guide you, for together we can make the world so much brighter.

Your light is needed and together we can shine and bloom and be happy and spread joy. Trust that you are safe always and dearly loved regardless of how things might appear at this moment.

Affirmation: "My life is unfolding in perfect ways."

27

Look deeper

If you are unsure whether you should take that next step, look deeper. If it feels too good to be true, look deeper. It is okay to look beyond the surface, to connect with your inner wisdom and make your decisions with caution. The better you feel about your next step, the greater your energy is when you proceed and the greater success you will receive. Trust in yourself. Trust in your guides and angels, and ask for only those who are of the highest light to be a part of your experience.

You are a magical person and you can manifest your intentions into reality. The clearer you feel, the faster you will see the results of your manifestations. The angels also wish to remind you to dream big, and don't settle for less than you desire. Serve in ways that bring you joy, for through that service, you also bring joy to others and they too will share their joy with us, and so on. Soon you will see a joyful world around you.

Affirmation: "I clearly see the truth and can easily discern the path before me."

28

See yourself and others through the eyes of the angels

Treat yourselves with unconditional love and acceptance always. Know that you might not be able to change some of the things in your life at this very moment; however you can change how you see and feel about that which you wish to change. And as you change how you see it, what you see often changes. Acceptance is the key.

Ask your angels for assistance, as they will immediately go to work on your behalf. They cannot help until you make your own choices and decisions and ask for their assistance. And, as you honour and follow the guidance of your heart, all that you desire will come your way.

Angel wisdom reminds you that you cannot change others, only yourself and how you see the world from your view. Have patience and trust; don't try to force things to happen. Allow the Universe to unfold as it should.

Be strong, for you are indeed stronger than you think you are, and your strength assures your desired outcome.

Affirmation: "I am strong and filled with compassionate love for all things. We are all a part of each other and filled with divine light. I unconditionally accept and love all things, regardless of how it appears."

29

Follow your heart

You have received some wonderful guidance as answers to your prayers. You've been receiving a message from your guardian angel that now is the time to follow your heart. Trust in the guidance you have been receiving, as it is a trustworthy message. Ask for and be open to receiving our support for anything that you need related to this desire. Positive new experiences are on the horizon, so now is the time to open up and follow what lies within your heart.

Expect the best. Wash away any negativity from your consciousness and past memories, and keep only the positive lessons and love. Don't hang on to anything that could weigh you down, such as resentment or bitterness. Let it go! Extract whatever teachings are needed and move on to a life of harmonious and peaceful actions.

Affirmation: "My heart is my guide and leads me where I want to go in love."

30

Time out

Take some time to just be in the moment, with no agenda or plan other than to be in the moment.

See the beauty that surrounds you. If you have difficulty finding the beauty from where you're at, look deeper. Take some deep breaths, close your eyes and relax. Ask that your heart chakra be opened and let your angels flood you with their love. Let that love pour all over you until every cell of your body is flooded with that beautiful energy and then let that love enfold you in an orb of love. And then, just enjoy that beautiful feeling. Feel the smile of bliss and let it fill you. When you are done, open your eyes and see the beauty that surrounds you in this new light. Have faith and hope, because something positive is on the horizon that perhaps you cannot see just yet. Trust that that is exactly where you are heading and keep taking the next step.

Affirmation:"I claim time and space for myself. I can feel more love and compassion each day. Everything on the earth carries a spark of the Divine within it. I can see these sparks more and more each day."

31

Spiritual awakening

We are helping you awaken your spiritual sight. Now is a great time to learn, study, and gather information. Enjoy being the student of life and open your heart to greater understanding and compassion. The angels wish to guide you to study the different aspects of your spiritual self for in the future, you will synthesize your knowledge and use it to help others in the creation of the new Earth.

As you expand your conscious understanding, those who are ready to awaken their spiritual gifts will be drawn to your light. Ask your angels to assist you and guide you to a teacher, a book, or a class. We are here to help you along the way. Our purpose is to serve humankind, and nothing brings us more bliss than to help you find yours. Quiet your mind and ask for us to enter and we will be your teachers and lead you to other humans who are best suited for your continued awakening.

Affirmation: "I am tuned in to my spiritual sight. I am grateful for this continued awakening, and each day it gets stronger and clearer."

32

Celebrate

Celebrate each moment. Celebrate the endings of each cycle in your life, for endings bring new beginnings. New opportunities, situations and relationships are built on the new foundation that you are creating for yourself. Change is inevitable. Rejoice, as your new spiritual experiences are changing the way you view yourself, others and the world. As you change your view of the world, the things you look at transform around you.

Allow your spiritual gifts to open. Ask your angels to assist in your transformation, and they will eagerly go to work on your behalf. The angels wish to remind you that they are bound by universal law of non-interference and we patiently wait for the human to request their help. We can guide you through study, prayer, and meditation, if you invite us into your experience.

The angels love for you is unconditional. Angel wisdom suggests for each one to also love each other unconditionally as love is giving, kind and patient. So open your heart and give your love.

Affirmation: "I am loving and giving. I am free."

33

Easy does it

There is no need to hurry or force things to happen. Everything is occurring as it should. Honour and follow your inner wisdom. Trust the guidance of your heart. As you trust and follow this guidance, prosperity in the area of your choosing will come your way.

Use the power of positive affirmations. Make little cards of the affirmations you desire and carry them with you. Place them on little notes around your home as reminders of states of being you desire to achieve. Believe that they are already here and with you, and open the gates of manifestation.

Be honest with yourself. Let your true nature shine through. As you do this others will see the beauty of your light and be brave enough to take those steps out of their darkness and follow the path of light. You are very deeply honoured for the courage in your heart as you step forward into your contracts. You are so dearly loved as the way-shower that you are for others as you create the new earth.

Affirmation: "Everything flows easily to me as I am ready and open to receive it."

34

Be flexible

Life is filled with change and surprises. Your angel guidance is to flow with the current, for it is resisting that flow which creates challenges. Ask your angels to help you open your mind and your heart to new ideas and fresh options. For you are indeed receiving trustworthy guidance and ideas as answers to your prayers. You can safely move forward with it, knowing that we are with you every step of the way. Please listen to and follow the steps we are communicating to you through your intuition, thoughts and especially your dreams.

We are particularly fond of communicating with you through your dreams. Ask each night for us to enter and communicate with you in your dreams and that if there is anything significant, that you intend to recall it when you awaken. And then in the morning ask "Did I dream?" and write down what you are remembering, even if it is vague. Then, when you have the time enter into a meditation and recall that dream, we will guide you back to what is important for you and guide you to the information that you seek.

Affirmation: "I recall the messages which are important to me. I am receiving trustworthy guidance that is of the highest light always."

35

Desire

What do you do desire? Angel wisdom suggests that you spend some time alone, preferably in nature, meditating about your desires and intentions. Ask the angels to help you gain a positive perspective. What do you desire right now? Visualize it, hold the vision without any doubt, and it will come.

Negativity will block your desires, as this cancels out your desired outcome. Remember, you get what you think about, so be very clear on what thoughts you hold.

Then, take action. Stay in touch with your truth. Trust your intuition and lovingly assert yourself. Stay committed to your vision. Revise it as necessary for your original desires can changes as you expand and move forward and see things in a different light. It is important for you to stay focused on your desires, yet it is also important to be true to your heart. If that desire should be happening in an outcome that doesn't feel or match your energy you think you are projecting, adjust it to be in line with your desired vibrations. Oftentimes what sounds good at the time is not really what you desire. Change it any time you desire something different.

Ask your angels for assistance and know that we are here and helping all those who ask, even if you don't see the tangible results yet.

Affirmation: "I no longer allow doubts or negative thoughts to stay in my mind. As soon as one comes my

way, I instantly replace it with something new and desirable."

36

Hope

Have faith and hope. There is something new on the horizon that perhaps you cannot see just yet. There is nothing to worry about. You are safe, and things really are under control and Divine providence. Faith is trust and trust is a powerful tool. Allow only positive thoughts and love into wherever you are. Love and emotions raise the vibration and ensure the highest outcome for the good of all. There is always another sunrise tomorrow.

Enjoy peace in your heart and trust. Give us any feelings of doubt, anger, resentment or blame. Give us any feelings of heaviness so we can lighten your load. Let us shroud your loving outlook. And feel the great love we have for you and infuse that love in all that you choose to create.

Affirmation: "I choose for my highest good and I trust that wonderful new options are coming my way."

37

Emerging to new heights

As you begin to emerge from your cocoon of spiritual growth, you will find that your expectations and standards of self have increased. Don't settle for less than you desire.

The changes that you are experiencing are divinely directed by your new born willingness to open your heart and mind to more love and guidance.

Your sensitivity increases with each expansion of your soul and spirit. Notice the loving guidance you hear inside your mind, as well as from other, as well as the messages that draw your attention, as this is how we often send messages to the human world. Trust your own inner knowingness; Trust your own connections, as this is part of the purpose of ascension, to empower you.

The angels remind you that they are here to serve and assist humanity, not do the journey for you. Our mission is to allow you your our own journey and expansion. We will not tell you how to do your journey, we support you as you do the journey, and your experiences and the way that you choose to approach your path assists in the growth of others and Universal energy of all that is.

Affirmation: "I am awakening more and more each day to a new way of being and doing that is in alignment with my higher purpose."

38

Magical

You are a magical being. You are a magical person who can manifest your clear intentions into reality. Ask your angels to help to light your way, for the brightness of clear intentions is such an easy path to follow. As you honour and follow the guidance of your heart and inner wisdom, prosperity will indeed come your way.

Pay attention to the thoughts and ideas that come to you, either through feelings, words, or actions, as these are answers to your prayers. Pay particular attention to those that come in three's for they are indeed the prompting of spirit. We are often repetitious in your suggestions for you, as the human doesn't always trust so easily. If you doubt it, then so shall it be, however if you embrace it and go forward with your next task, so shall that be. Whatever your intention, so shall it be your reality. Therefore, focus on that which you desire, and it shall be.

Affirmation: "I am focused on my visions. I listen to the guidance of my inner wisdom and spirit. I am tapped in at all times and trust the messages that come through my heart."

39

You are powerful

It is safe for you to be powerful. You are powerful and you know how to be powerful in loving ways that benefit others as well as yourself. Be your powerful self with compassion.

Your angel guidance is to connect to your still, quiet center and listen to the wisdom of your soul. Then make your decisions, thoughts, and words from your own infinite self. You are safe always.

With this newfound connection to your wisdom, life takes on a new perspective, as dramas and fears become insignificant in comparison with the magnificence of the overall picture. As you see the world from this perspective, wonderful new experiences are now on the horizon.

Enjoy life from the perspective of love. Use your powers for your highest good and therefore the highest good of all.

Affirmation: "I am powerful. I use power with love and create the life I desire."

40

Open your heart to love

The more you allow yourself to love, the greater depth and meaning your life holds.

Everything you desire and every prayer that you seek comes as a result of opening your heart to both sending and receiving love. Love is vital to life. Release any fears and transform them with love.

Your heart is the gateway of receptivity. It is the answer to every question you have about your love life, relationships, health, life purpose, and so forth. Be more loving to yourself for others will treat you as you see and treat yourself.

Your angel guidance is to open your heart and count your blessings. Say thank you from your heart. Whenever you say thank you, more is bestowed upon you.

Affirmation:"I am grateful for everything in my life. My heart is open."

41

Dream big

Let go of any small thoughts for yourself and others. See yourself succeeding in any endeavour that you choose to focus on. Imagine it as happening in the most grandest of fashion, even bigger and more elaborate that you can possibly imagine. As you do this, remember the exhilarating feeling and carry that energy with you. Every time you think of that desire, or take a step towards it, invoke that feeling.

Send positive thoughts for the changes that you seek as well as the fulfillment of your wishes. Ask the angels for help and they will fan the sparks of potential and bring them to life. Let your angels work on the details while you focus on the joy of having along the way.

Be at peace regardless. Angel wisdom reminds you that you can hover in the eye of any hurricane that may swirl around you right now. Through breath and intention, you can stay centered regardless of what's happening in your life. This inner foundation of peace has a very powerful healing effect. As this happens, your outer life begins to reflect your inner one. Be at peace to ensure a peaceful outcome.

Affirmation: "I am at peace; I bring a new tranquility to my life and to a smoother road ahead. I am eternally optimistic. I deserve the grandest life."

42

A new day dawning

Each day is a new day. Live each day as if it were your last one. Give hugs and love to those you care about. Smile and let them feel your love for them and for life. Aspire to oneness each day with all of humanity. Feel the beauty and the love that all the weaves that Mother Earth has to share and how every rock, tree or insect plays a vital role in your evolution.

You are safe and protected from all types of harm. Relax and feel safe on your human journey. Angel wisdom reminds you that it is each person's responsibility to keep these beautiful weaves protected and honoured. Love is the answer. The vibration of your love for each other and all things is truly what makes a difference. Now is the perfect time to act on your inspirations in sharing that love.

Seek out those with knowledge and experience, yet also trust your own heart and the inner wisdom in all things, in each step that you take, for it is about how each of you lives your lives and do your journey. See life with the unconditional love that your guides, angels and ancestors have for you, your success (and you are successful, regardless how you view life on your side of the veil), and you are dearly loved for all that you do.

Affirmation: "I offer my love and compassion to all those who are a part of this earth experience."

43

Just for today follow your bliss

Take some time from your day to do something for yourself. Choose something that truly feeds your heart. It can be a 30 minute segment of dancing to music, a walk in the park, spending some special time with a loved one, flying a kite, or whatever else you can think of that brings you 30 minutes of pure, heartfelt joy. For it is after these moments in time that you feel closer to your life purpose, feel clear minded and are closer to our vibration and are more able to hear the whisperings of spirit.

Take some time from your busy day and just be in joy and in love with yourself for at least 30 minutes and allow whatever inspirations come your way to unfold before you, for as you honour and follow your inner guidance from your heart, the more abundant your experience becomes.

Affirmation: "I do activities each day that bring me joy."

44

Truth and integrity

Live your truth with integrity. For these two actions lead to the serenity that is so desired. The angels suggest that now is the time to take action towards being in your truth. Begin to live your life from your truth, no one else's. And worry not about how they live their life; focus your attention on your life and what you want to create for yourself. Worry not how others see you, for that is their issue. We are not saying to ignore others; we are saying to love each other for who they are, regardless. Honour them for the choices they make in their journey, regardless if you would do it differently. Honour yourself for the choices you have made, even if it seems you might have gone off the path at times. It is those side journeys that assist your growth and expansion, and helps you gain great insight and clarity as you go on your path.

There is no 'one path' for anyone. There are all kinds of choices and different routes to take along the way. Look where you are at today and be thankful for all that led you this place, regardless! Acceptance means unconditional love. Accept everyone exactly as they are, without judging, blaming or wanting to change them, this includes how you see yourself as well.

Live in your truth with great integrity, trust your inner wisdom and lovingly go forward.

Affirmation: "I live my life from my truth and integrity."

45

Divine passion

Be honest with yourself. What is your heart's true desire? Look deep within your heart and find what it is that creates Divine passion within you. Eliminate power struggles, conflicts and competition as these stem from the egos desire to win. Cooperate with others for the highest good of all as this promotes harmony and togetherness and draws the very best from everyone.

Keep charging ahead, bring people together and explore how you can mutually assist each other. Expect miraculous solutions to appear. We will guide you on how you can create abundance in all things. We can work together to create that which is your true passion.

Affirmation: "I co create with everyone. Together we are stronger and there is enough for everyone to have everything that they desire."

46

Divine magic

Expect miracles; this opens the doorway for them to enter your life. Now is the time to take charge of your creations, for you are surrounded in extra magical energy. Your manifestation ability is heightened. Use this time to focus upon your desires.

It is time for you to take charge and assume your role as your true radiant, powerful and intelligent self. Make decisions instead of passively waiting for opportunities to emerge. Give yourself permission to do what feels right. If you are unsure what you truly want, ask for Divine guidance through prayer, meditation, or ritual. The Universe responds to your vibration. When you are clear about your aims and intentions you see more of the results you desire.

The angels will support you, as you have the power to heal and alter the course of your life.

Affirmation: "I vibrate to attract miracles in my life each day."

47

Moon power

Notice how the change in the moon affects your energy and manifestations. As you pay attention to the moon's cycles, you can capitalize on the gifts she offers. As you approach your next full moon, prepare your crystals for clearing and recharging.

As well, the angels want us to remember that humans are also affected by this energy and suggest that a meditation for clearing and recharging yourselves at this time is also optimal. You are a powerful being and you know how to be powerful in loving ways that assists others through the example that you set.

Use the amazing energy the moon has to offer to recharge your energy also. Feel the magnificence that is shared during this powerful time and find a quiet place for contemplation and look within on the days leading up to the full moon to utilize its full power. Ask your angels to help to guide you if you are unsure of the best way to utilize this beautiful and free resource. Ask your angels to enfold you in their angel wings and provide you with a safe haven in which to relax and re center yourself.

Affirmation: "I recharge and renew with the phases of the moon."

48

Detach from drama

Surround situations in your life with a loving light. As you expand and heal yourself and become lighter and more sensitive to your environments, you will find that you are more receptive to the emotions of others and therefore feel this energy in a different way. Since humans evolve at different rates, there are is usually a variety of issues and dramas taking place. When you find yourself in situations that include others sharing their stories with you, infuse the conversation with loving light as they share with you, smile and listen.

Do not offer your counsel unless expressly asked for, just send them loving light. Most often others share to gain their own clarity. As you become a more compassionate being, open yourself up to more compassion, but most of all access the wisdom within that recognizes the Divine in everyone and everything and all that is. This action spreads much light, joy, and freedom and is an energy that empowers others.

Affirmation: "I am safe and protected in all ways. I am filled with greater and greater compassion each day and I have greater awareness and love for others and my connection to all things."

49

Perfect timing

Now is the perfect moment to act on your inspirations. New doors are opening at this time. There is something positive on the horizon that perhaps you can't see yet, so please don't give up just before it arrives. Have faith and trust that all things are currently as they should be. Take a step each day that leads you closer to that which you desire. Don't delay or procrastinate, as all the ingredients are ripe and ready for your success. Are you ready? Be brave and know that we are always by your side.

Take some time out of your busy schedule and find some moments of serenity. When you become deeply serene and still, you connect to the higher powers of the Universe, and have access to Divine guidance and your path in life becomes smooth and free flowing. Let us hold you in serenity and grace.

Affirmation: "I am in a state of grace and serenity and flow with the Universal energy. I am always in the right place at the right time."

50

Kindness

Open your heart to the gentle qualities of caring and compassion. Be kind to yourself. Be gentle with yourself. Cherish yourself. When you do something for yourself, you automatically extend that same energy to others. Every cell in your body will tingle with joy as you begin to treat yourself with kindness. Love yourself.

Ask your angels for help if you are unsure how to make the life changes that allow for you to be more kind to yourself. Know that kindness is part of your Divine life purpose.

We are behind you every step of the way, offering our love, you strength and courage. Quiet yourself and listen carefully to your angels, feel us and the love that we have for you. Part of our Divine purpose is Overlight you, support you and to always be here for you.

Affirmation: "I am filled with love and compassion for everyone including myself."

51

Take charge

Life's circumstances can be healed with gentle love, yet there is also a need for strength and truthfulness.

It is possible to be both assertive and angelic at the same time. Call upon the angels for courage and guidance when you need to speak your truth. With practice, this becomes easier and second nature. These are opportunities for personal and spiritual growth.

First, decide what you want. Be clear about the conditions that are acceptable and unacceptable for you. The universe responds when you are clear about your aims and intentions. Talk openly and honestly about your feelings. Be the resolute warrior in your life. The angels are working behind the scenes to help you, even if you don't yet see the results. Trust in your own power to heal and create anew.

Angel wisdom reminds you to recognize who you truly are, an evolving, powerful spiritual being. Align with your true power and nature and watch your spirit soar.

Affirmation: "I am aligned with my true power. I communicate my thoughts easily and with love, always."

52

Divine order

Everything is how it needs to be right now. Look past the illusions and notice the underlying order. Know that you are never alone and that we are with you always and in all ways. Of course we must always be asked to assist, however we are always there. Be patient and know that your dreams will happen and things will always be changing, evolving to another level of light and love. Be at peace with the process and keep doing your journey, joyfully.

Find the joy and the gift in all things and where you are at this time. Look beyond the surface and seek light in the heart of every person. Delight in everything, for joy is a key to enlightenment.

Affirmation: "I find joy all around me. I accept that everything is in Divine order and therefore as it should be right now."

53

Light

Focus your light on your desired outcome. As your light becomes stronger and clearer, a happy outcome will happen in the very near future. Ask your angels to fill you with more light, for it contains spiritual information and wisdom. These are keys to the Universe and bring love and peace, as well as unlocking the wisdom within you.

Let your light shine on all your creations and surround them with positive expectations. Have patience and faith; don't try to force things to happen, just let them unfold as they should for the good of all. Rest, relax and enjoy the process of creation, for it is that is truly your purpose.

Affirmation: "I am Light."

54

Endings

The old must be released so that the new can enter. Just like the beautiful trees that surround your earth that lose their leaves each year, it is time to shed that which no longer serves you. Are there unreleased situations and people that you have not let go of yet?

Life is a cycle of beginnings and endings. Each completion makes way for new thoughts, people and events to enter. New growth emerges where it has room to grow.

Take a moment today and spend some time in contemplation, preferably in nature and see the wonders of the cycles of life. Nature trusts that the sun will rise tomorrow and the spring will come, bringing with it new growth and life. This is the time for rest and rejuvenation before the next cycle begins. While in nature write a letter from your angels or guides asking 'what is it that I need to release' and watch as the answers come to you. Don't analyze or second guess them now, just write from your heart. And then later read your letter, and see if there is anything you are holding onto that needs to be transformed.

Enjoy the process, as this is indeed the process of evolution and that is what you came to earth to experience.

Affirmation: "Just as I see the cycles all around me, I recognize and appreciate the cycles in my life."

55

Worthiness

Know that you are worthy. Angel wisdom reminds you that you deserve to receive good in all ways and always. Stay optimistic as your dreams will come true. You are making steady progress, although it doesn't always seem to be quick enough at the time. Don't give up before the miracles begin to occur all around you.

To increase the flow in your prosperity, call upon us to assist you. We are always here and available. We are never too busy and are not governed by time and space and you are.

Remember to bring love into your daily activities. As you become more love, your every thought, feeling and actions are a unique contribution to humankind and this evolving journey that is occurring in your dimension of time and space. And these ripple out into other dimensions in undreamed of ways.

Affirmation: "I choose to find love in all things and situations. I am flowing in a steady stream of peace and love at all times."

56

Empowerment

Your personal power increases the more you trust and love yourself. It is time to utilize and step into your role as an ambassador of Light and Love.

You are a powerful co-creator of Divine energy, and it is safe for you to be that powerful being. Ask the angels to assist you in realizing and releasing any thoughts, feelings and situations that hold you back from taking your role in creating that which you desire. This allows for new thoughts, ideas and inspirations to come your way.

Angel wisdom suggests that you take a moment each day and focus on your strengths, next focus on clearing and stabilizing your energy fields, then, focus on the characteristics you want to foster and grow. When you feel strong, powerful and balanced, it is easier to focus on the goals and dreams you would like to create right now. Imagine them as if you already have what you desire and that they are a part of your vibration. Use your power with wisdom and joy.

Then, enjoy the shifts you see around you, and use your power to create a better world for yourself, and others.

Affirmation:" I am a powerful creator force in the service of Light and Love."

57

Longing for home

Sometimes there is a longing for the peace and love of home, and many of you wish to be back in the loving embrace of the Creator.

Your angels would like to remind you that home is within your heart and that is why you long to back in the loving light of the Divine. And, while we await your return after a journey well done, we also know that your soul always wants to grow and expand, and when you are here with us you so desire to come into another experience and continue your journey.

Those who have come back to join are safe and love you. If you feel sadness about this illusionary separation, call upon your angels and deceased loved ones and they will be there to comfort, support and love you, just as they have always been. A conscious visit with a loved one can do wonders to lift your spirit.

Feel your heart and feel the love and you are once again home.

Affirmation: "I can feel the love of home within me."

58

Adventure

Life is an adventure. Be ready for the unexpected and make the most of all opportunities.

The angel wisdom suggests you get out of any habits or ruts if you are feeling stuck. Do things that are different and face life with a sense of wonder, just as you did as a child.

If the path ahead seems dark and scary, do as you would if you were exploring a dark place, shine your light. Ask your angels to light up the way. Then watch for the signs and signals that tell you where to go next. The light on the path in front of you may not go far ahead, however you will see enough to guide your way.

Explore the new with excitement and courage. These magnetic qualities attract money and career opportunities and add zest to your life and relationships. Embrace the changes that come your way, and go beyond what is comfortable for you, for this is how your spirit grows.

The angels are encouraging you to move forward with anticipation, expectancy, gratitude and hope and to look for the joy within each step you take.

Affirmation:"I am eager for life's adventures."

59

Decisions

Should I go this way or that way?

Some days you are completely sure of your decisions, the next day you are not. Angel wisdom reminds you to ask yourself "Does this path lead me closer to my Divine purpose?" even if you aren't sure of what that purpose is.

Be patient, as the easiest route isn't necessarily the one that leads you where you want to go. Trust that you are exactly where you need to be and find the peace that lies within. Finding the peace within yourself regardless of where you are leads to decisions made with a stronger foundation. Does this decision bring you more peace? If you are still unsure, ask your angels to assist you. We are always here to help to guide you where you want to go.

When you make your decision, then you can focus energy upon that choice whether you are working on relationships, work, a journey or anything else in your life. We can see the light of your commitment and are better able to energize it as well. When no decision is made, we are not sure of where you want to go and then put more choices before you in our attempts to assist you. If you are still not sure which way to go, focus on joyful service where you are at this time and new ideas will come your way when the time is right.

Affirmation: "I am at peace and filled with joy with each step that I take."

60

Positive change

Your likes and dislikes are changing, and you are outgrowing situations that once appealed to you. These are all positive signs that signal spiritual growth. Some of these situations are easy to let go of, while others are a blessing in disguise. These are the ones that push you into making positive changes in your life. Going beyond your comfort zone is what helps you grow and transform.

Your angels stand ready to support you with whatever you ask. Let go of the past and enjoy the ride. This is truly what you have been longing to do.

Take very good care of yourself through these changes. Withdraw if you need to. This is a time for dreams, magic, and a little solitude. Keep moving forward at a steady pace and tidy up loose ends along the way. You will be glad you did as these activities will create the energetic flow of creativity that you require.

Angel wisdom reminds you to say no to anything that diverts you from your path. Let go of any procrastinations and perfectionism's, and break your major goals into smaller steps and then take one step at a time.

Affirmation: "Change signals new growth in my life. I eagerly step forward into whatever is next on my path."

61

New dawn

Endings are always followed by new beginnings. Sometimes it is difficult to let the old go for fear that it will either not be replaced, or something you don't want might come your way.

Change is not always easy; however it is the catalyst that brings about the evolution of you and your desires. Call upon your angels to comfort, and to guide you to the next step. Happiness awaits you in ways that you cannot imagine.

It is important for you to express your feelings during these times of transitions. Keep a journal, talk to a trusted friend or adviser, or you can discuss everything with your angels. The more that you can release, the freer you feel and completions always makes way for the new that you desire to enter into your life. After all, isn't that what you have been asking for?

We are always, always here to lend you courage and support, give you angel hugs that allow you to feel safe until the time comes that you feel the confidence to emerge into the new beautiful you.

Affirmation: "I welcome each new dawn for it brings with it a fresh new experience."

62

Perfect timing

Now is the perfect time to act on your inspirations. Yes, the timing is right for you to follow the passion that lies within your heart. Hold positive thoughts and expectations as you set your intent to the Universe. Call upon your angels for strength and direction. We can assist you by removing any negativity and to become open minded, clear and wise. Connect with your inner wisdom as you focus upon your desires and follow the steps that are put before you. A happy outcome follows your positive expectations.

As you travel through life you have learned valuable lessons that have prepared you for the next steps in your journey. Take bold steps, while listening to the wise guidance of your heart as you move forward in your truth and your passion. Trust that it is now time to reap the rewards for your patience and all the work you have done that has brought you here now.

Affirmation: "I am guided by my inspirations."

63

Contemplation time

Spend some time alone each day meditating. Take some time out of your busy schedule to take care of yourself. This includes some introspection upon where you are, and where you would like to go. Creating a regular practice of taking time out to nurture yourself will keep your energy high and your thoughts clear. So many of you beautiful Lightworkers are giving so much of yourself to others, it is important to take a time out and be sure that your needs are being met on all levels. Ask your angels to assist you if you need help finding some alone time each day to nourish your spirit, nourish your physical vessel, clear your mind and get clear on your focus and to feed and love your emotional body.

As you continue your path of awakening it is important to make that special time for yourself. It allows for you to find the homeostasis that is necessary as your emerging continues. The physical body is the densest of all the bodies and it requires a little time to catch up with your growth. Honour yourself and your process, for it is you who are the ones that help so many others begin their path of awakening, as you step forward into merging your spirit self with your physical self and walk the path of light.

Affirmation: "I take time to honour myself and my process. I am emerging and evolving each day, shedding the old and welcoming the new energy that surrounds me as I continue to become a human of light."

64

You are supported

You deserve the best. Reach for the stars with your dreams and desires, and don't compromise. You are surrounded by loving support always. Each of you has a bevy of angels and guides who love and support you.

Quiet your mind and your body and feel our love. Ask for us to assist and we are always willing, able and ready. Pay attention to the synchronicities around you, for there is truly no such thing as chance. These are carefully orchestrated occurrences set up by your higher self and your entourage to create the opportunities that you have requested.

Explore your options and possibilities as it is a good time for change. Change is evolution.

Take your inner child outside to play, as this freedom opens your mind and heart to our connection and you can more clearly see the possibilities that are available to you. As well, it brings you joy, and that is one of the most powerful forces in the Universe.

Feel our love, affection and attention. Let us nurture you this day.

Affirmation: "I feel the love and support that surrounds me and helps me reach my goals."

65

Simplify your life

Has your energy has been fragmented? Perhaps it's time for an adjustment.

Angel wisdom suggests it is time to take drastic measures to simply your life. This means clearing your home of unnecessary items, cancelling subscriptions to extraneous publications, saying no to demands on your time, getting organized, and being more efficient with respect to your schedule.

You may feel that such a project is overwhelming. However if you take one day a week to whittle down the clutter, you'll feel an enormous lifting of weight from your soul. Or perhaps a little each day, which ever feels more comfortable. This results in an energy and esteem boost that will enable you to complete the tasks at hand. Your soul, mind and body will thank you for your simpler life!

Clearing out the physical 'things' in your life helps to clear the mental clutter and assists you in finding or gaining clarity. It helps you feel more free and lighter, so take some time to simplify your physical world and enjoy the freedom it brings your way.

Affirmation: "I easily attract all that I need into my life; I therefore no longer need to hang on to the things in my life."

66

Clear intentions

Be clear about your desires, and focus upon them with truth, trust and passion. Now is the perfect moment for you to act on your inspirations. The doors are open, while you walk through them with the angels at your side.

Everyone and everything is on your side, supporting your desired outcome. Don't procrastinate, as all the ingredients are ripe for your success. Allow yourself to imagine that your desires are already manifested and experience the emotional and physical feelings of those manifested desired.

Your angel guidance is to welcome the new in your life. If you are unsure what is the next best step for you to take, consult an expert. Once that first step is taken towards your desires, the Universe then gives additional help. Seek wise counsel from someone who has expertise in this area, and benefit from their knowledge and experience. To attract the right expert to assist you, be it an earthy being or your angels and guides, set your intentions and ask that they be drawn to you.

Affirmation: "A helpful knowledgeable, experienced and wise being with integrity is in my life right now, and available to assist me."

And then, be open to the signs, take notes, and give thanks. Then, enjoy the results of your creations.

67

Listening and receiving

You are receiving trustworthy guidance. We are leading you toward the answer to your prayers. Be open to receiving Divine guidance and assistance. Please listen to follow the steps we are communicating through your intuition, thoughts, and dreams.

You are filled with wonderful ideas, these are real and trustworthy. You can safely move forward, knowing that we are by your side every step of the way.

Quiet your body and your mind dear ones, and from that deep, still place within you, hear and feel us. Learn to trust with little things and move up from there if this is at all a task. Be patience with yourself.

Affirmation: "I easily hear and understand the messages from my angels and higher self."

68

Support of the Universe

Trust that you have the support of the Universe at your fingertips. Developing this powerful quality will help you move mountains.

Surround yourself with positive energy and positive people, as this will assist you in gaining trust in the possibility of all things that are available to you. Put your trust in yourself and your ability to tap into the power of higher powers that surround you in all ways, always. Pray with integrity from your still, wise center and know that your requests are heard and answered.

As you experience and adjust to the changes that are happening in your life, know that this energy of discovery is like an adventure to a new land, filled with awe and hope. Release any mental energy that is holding you in the past so you can follow your path to the happy outcomes you desire.

Your angel guidance is to increase your trust in the Infinite Universal energy that is available to all who choose to tap into it.

Affirmation:"I know that I am supported by the Universe."

69

Make a wish

There is magical energy all around you. You are surrounded by magical energy all the time, regardless as to what others would have you believe. We tell you it is always there for your creations. So, make a wish today, then, state out loud that which you desire to create. *Feel* the *essence* of that which you wish to create and what it will bring into your life.

Awaken the God/Goddess within you through dance, music, self-care, and appreciating your Divinity. See the Divinity with yourself. See the love, compassion, grace and wisdom that you have within yourself and then go out and see that Divinity in others and all things.

You deserve the best! Reach for the stars with your dreams and desires. Bring those desires onto your psychical plane by taking action each day that fills you joy and is part of your passion. Allow the magical energy around you to assist in your creations. Be patient with yourself. Love yourself as we love and honour you.

Take a deep breath, what is your dream, then begin the feelings of joy and watch as the energy takes off and explodes all around you like rockets of desire.

Affirmation: "I see love and gifts all around me."

70

Trust

Have hope and trust that new things are on the horizon. You may not fully see the formations yet, however if you have spent some time meditating and day dreaming about what it feels like to have these desires in your life, they will soon materialize.

Set your intent on something you truly desire to create in your life (this can also be an emotion like love). When you can feel the pure focus of your thought, call upon your entourage of light beings, and trust that you are worthy, it will surely come your way.

In the meantime while you are waiting for the fruition of your dreams, focus on using your talents and your skills for the common good. Do things that bring you joy and therefore joy to those around you. Promote harmony and togetherness. Feel the sense of a job well done, and share your love with all that you meet.

See yourself how we see you, as a pure light of the essence of the Divine.

Affirmation: "I trust in the energy of the Universe."

71

Finding the gifts

Your angel guidance is to find a quiet space and look within. Take time and space to review your life. Take time and space for yourself to recuperate from life's challenges, to reflect on the way ahead, to strengthen yourself and to prepare for the next phase of your life.

In this time, find the blessings and gifts within each situation. This can be a very emotional experience and very cleansing, so ask for us to be by your side for comfort and love, as well, if you need our help in seeing the gifts within the moment, we are here to ease that burden too.

It is time to release and see all things with unconditional love and acceptance. New beginnings are on their way!

Affirmation:"I see myself and others through Angels' eyes; I see love and know all is perfect."

72

Surround yourself, situations, and people with loving energy and light

If you are unsure of what to do next, take a pause and surround yourself with a loving pink and blue light, then surround the situation with the same light, then engulf all of the people involved with that same loving, peaceful and balanced light. Look deep into your heart, and then deeper into the situation. Feel love and understanding to all involved in the highest light of love, then proceed further as you feel more balanced and stronger.

Let the beautiful waves of the ocean speak to your soul, soothing and healing you. Cleansing and clearing, then leaving you treasures upon the shores with each exhale. Take the time you need, and then take the action that you feel guided to take. Trust that you are always supported and cared for.

Affirmation: "I surround myself and those I love with loving, calm and peaceful light."

73

Focus on serenity and kindness

Your soul desires only to be joyful and to serve the evolution of itself and therefore humanity.

In order to be kind you must open your heart to the gentle qualities of caring and compassion, Serenity bestows inner peace, tranquility and calmness of mind. These two qualities bring joy into your life. Joy is of the highest vibrating energy.

When you feel serene, you are your own person, for nothing and no one can bother, upset or influence you. Be kind to yourself. Have reasonable expectations and give yourself much due praise. Nurture the gentle quality of kindness and cherish yourself. As you become deeply serene and still, you become connected to the higher vibrating energy of the Universe. This energy is your connection to Divine guidance and tapping into this stream of wisdom can illuminate your path in life and the journey becomes smooth and flowing.

Delight in everything, for joy is a key to enlightenment. Your rewards will be a sense of inner peace, warmth and love.

Affirmation:"I find joy in everything. I am serene and peaceful."

74

Day dreams

You can more easily hear and receive our messages through daydreaming. Relax and open your mind to receiving, without directing your thoughts. Just let the information flow and notice the feelings, visions, or ideas as if you were watching a movie. When you are done with this visualization, write in a journal about the information that you have received. All that you receive in that short time is recorded in your mind. Just take the time to write it down to look at later.

Remember, happy outcomes follow positive expectations. Have patience and trust, and don't try to force things to happen. Relax, and be in a state of joy.

Affirmation: "I see happy outcomes for all that I desire."

75

Release

It is time to release and trust that you are worthy. It is time to release old memories, habits, thoughts and mental patterns which hold you in a lower vibration. Let us angels help you to bring order, discipline, joy, and clarity into your life so that everything begins to run more smoothly.

Trust that your prayers are indeed manifesting. Remain positive and follow your inner guidance. And remember to play and enjoy yourself along the way. We are often more able to get messages to you when you play with the wild abandon of a child. In that state, you are clear of the things that bog you down and are more open to all things wonderful, magical and possible in your life. And you return to the world renewed, refreshed, and with a new perspective and heightened awareness.

Affirmation: "I happily release thoughts, habits and memories that no longer serve my growth."

76

Trust

Trust in the support of the Universe. As you honour and trust the guidance of your heart, the more of your dreams come true. Be it a new home or place of employment. Movement towards positive focused thoughts ushers in new positive energy for you to work with.

Use common sense and discernment and do not give your power up to another. Trust in yourself and the support and love that you feel from entourage of light beings.

Your angel guidance is to increase your trust in the Infinite and in yourself.

Affirmation: "I have faith in the support of the Universe, and in my ability to create my desires in the physical world."

77

Reach for the stars

You deserve the best. Reach for the stars with your dreams and your desires. Hold steadfast in your focus of those desires and trust the divine guidance that is helping you along the way.

Be magnanimous, see the good in others and give them the benefit of the doubt, always. Forgive yourself. Open up to compassion, but most of all access the wisdom within you that recognizes the Divine in everything and everyone. With this energy you are not only open to receiving; you are offering others your grace.

This energy offers you a smoother road ahead and a beautiful new tranquility. Everything is possible in this incredible Universe. Set your sights and then be open to however spirit brings it your way.

Affirmation: "I follow my heart and do what I love each moment."

78

Love yourself

You are a most beautiful being of light. As is every other human, animal, mineral, you are all made of that same spark of Divinity, each and every one of you and everything. Each one of you is on a journey. For each of you that do this journey is on a different path and sometimes they touch, and sometimes they cross, and sometimes they stay together for a long, long time, appearing as one, then they too separate and move on. Each of you is searching for love and joy in your own way. Bless each other, bless yourself, and move on.

Pay attention to the signs on your journey; let others pay attention to their lane, pay attention to yours, even if you can see that their road looks more smoothly paved.

Unless asked, just honour their process for it is theirs, and focus upon your road and what you would like along the way. It is like those video games where people can build their own city and lives and those they interact with. Begin to trust that you too can create like that in your own life and focus on your own journey. For as you do this, you shift the other reality potentials for all the others that are here playing their game of life.

You change the potentials for each others as you begin to see love in yourself and then in all others. Release any judgements and just love unconditionally.

Affirmation: "My focus is on my path of Light and what is best for me."

79

Move forward

It is time to move forward. It is time to let go of the old and worn out, so that the new can come in. As you are releasing the old, it is important to consciously choose what you want to create next.

This will lessen the lag time between, lessen the ups and the down, and bring you balance and harmony as you move along. As the old moves away and new begins to enter, keep charging ahead, don't take no for an answer, and expect miraculous solutions to appear before you.

To bring in a flow of new and fresh ideas, go outside and play like children. Children offer us a tremendous gift of joyfulness through playing. Join some kids at the park or play by yourself. The most important part is to just have some fun. Be in that joyous state and get some fresh air to clear out the cob webs.

Affirmation: "I am ready, eager and willing to move forward in my life."

80

Answered prayers

Your prayers are being heard beloved ones, and they are also being answered. The angels are working behind the scenes to help you, even if you don't see the results of this action. Know and trust that we have heard your prayers and are working by your side creating for you and with you to bring about your desires. Pay attention to the signs we send your way. Perhaps you receive an intuitive feeling or a new opportunity appears, or a book falls off the shelf. The angels often answer prayers by giving ideas or information in these everyday ways.

Angel wisdom reminds you that you will more easily hear and receive our messages if you daydream regularly. Relax and open your mind to receiving, without directing your thoughts. Just notice any feelings, visions, or ideas as if you were watching a movie. This is the seat of your creativity.

Affirmation: "My prayers are always answered and I clearly understand the messages I receive."

81

Grounding yourself

Your attention and work are needed upon the earth. When you spend too much time detached from the awareness of bodies, and the physical world, you can become ungrounded. It is important to remember that you are here to have a physical experience and regular connections to the Mother Earth will assist you in accomplishing the tasks you desire on the earth plane.

Your angel guidance is to regularly connect with mother earth during your meditation times. Connect with the plants, the animals and the minerals after doing any intense spiritual pursuits. Ask your angels to help you balance the spiritual and material worlds so that you can enjoy a fulfilling earthly journey.

Affirmation: "I regularly connect with the earth and feel the wonderful energy that is given back to me."

82

Discernment

Discernment sensing what feels right, and trusting that feeling, determining what feels right and brings value to your life.

Your angel guidance is to look deeper at all the relationships, people and situations in your life right now and responding with your inner feelings.

Feelings that come from inside like the quiet voice within you that says, "Don't do that", or "Don't go there", or "Follow that feather and see where it lands" or perhaps even, "Say hello and smile at that person". These are all promptings of your inner being, your spirit self that is always connected to your physical self. As you look deeper into your relationships, see the love that underlies all of them. Let that love be your guide.

Use discernment in all that you do. Take the gift offered from everything that you do, read and see. If you are reading or listening to something that doesn't feel right, send it love. If it feels completely wrong to you, politely smile and excuse yourself from the situation. If you can't leave it at that moment, take a few deep breaths, feel yourself surrounded by love and just be in the moment. Take in only that which resonates to you in that moment, and just leave the rest. It might be helping others at levels that are not a part of your journey.

Affirmation: "I trust and am tuned into what is right and brings value to my life at all times."

83

Change

It is okay to be nervous about change. Trust that when you walk through the gateway to the other side of everything, that a beautiful garden awaits you, even if it doesn't look so at the time. Some of the scariest of gateways leads to the most rich and exhilarating experiences. Be brave and know that we are always at your side, even if you don't feel it yet. Trust and believe and don't be swayed by the mental energy of failure from yourself or others. Ignore the sceptics and naysayers, and perhaps even try to avoid them for awhile while you get your sure footing once again.

Stay on your course with purposeful action, trust yourself, be yourself and follow your heart. Everything is lined up for your success, and change means that the new can enter, and that you are expanding and evolving your light.

Affirmation: "Change signifies that my life is expanding and new opportunities are coming my way."

84

Acknowledgement

Examine and note your gifts, talents and achievements. Look after yourself by acknowledging your desires and needs and then taking steps to meet them. When you accept all aspects of yourself, you feel more centered, grounded and confident. Then you can genuinely acknowledge the divineness of others. Become aware of and nurture the good qualities of the people in your life as well as in yourself. This brings out those qualities when you are together and you each begin to see each other in a new light.

Angel wisdom reminds you to recognize who you truly are, an evolved spirit in a human body. When you acknowledge your spiritual dimensions, you will align with your true self and together your spirit will soar. See the beautiful light that we see when we look at you and share that light with the world.

Affirmation:"I acknowledge the beauty of who I truly am."

85

Opportunity

Seize the day as something new is now available to you. It is up to you to use this opportunity to your greatest advantage. Be alert, be aware, and be prepared. Expect to see the signs that are put before you without any doubt that they will be there. Ask your angels and your inner guidance to be alert and to help you receive valuable information that will assist you on your path. Expect miraculous solutions to appear.

Spend time alone each day and meditate upon what you truly desire to create in your life. Visualize it as already with you and how that feels. Don't request how this comes about, only that it does, and leave the "how to's" up to us.

Know that you and your loved ones are safe and protected by your angels. We are always with you and you are never alone. We offer our gratitude to you for all that you do and support you always.

Affirmation: "I seize each opportunity that assists me in realizing my dreams and desires."

86

Purpose

There is no such thing as an accident or coincidence. Everyone and every situation are placed on your path for a purpose. Co incidents are carefully planned out occurrences of seemingly random events.

Your angel guidance is to ask your angels to help you find the purpose within your current path. It may be to strengthen you, or offer you an opportunity to resolve or forgive something or someone from the past. It can be to release old patterns, or simple to bring more happiness and joy into your life.

Ultimately the purpose for most of your experiences is to bring more joy, satisfaction and fulfillment into your life, although it doesn't always feel that way when you are going through a particularly trying time. Seek the soul qualities of that which you desire like laughter, joy, balance. This will help to place you on the path to your destiny. So, you are reminded to keep at it for it may be that new doors are opening for you as you find the gift within each experience.

Affirmation: "I am strong and determined. I am focused and also filled with joy and purpose."

87

Developing your senses

Take the time to notice and work on your abilities to hear, see and feel the loving guidance that we send your way.

Listen with your mind, heart and body, as we send you messages through all of these senses including earth angels in physical form. Your angel guidance is to develop and focus on using your different senses during your meditation practice. It is through consciously focusing on one area that it will improve and pick up the more subtle vibrations that are around you.

As well as the messages and signs we provide for you, we also send other humans to pass on messages. Look for repetitive signs before you. What catches your attention in the 3D world? If you notice a pattern, take that thought back into meditation with us and dialogue with us to help you gain a greater understanding.

The perfect time is now. There is no better time than today to begin a new spiritual practice of tuning into your own beautiful wisdom, and as you gain mastery in that area, tune in with another sense and keep moving forward. As you practice and perfect your skills, you become that conscious creator in your life.

Affirmation:"Each day I become better and better at sensing the messages from my guides and angels."

88

Action

Ready, set, go

Now is the perfect time to move forward and work towards your goals and dreams. Even the slightest movement towards those desires brings about energy that affects everything in its wake. Imagine if you were to put a lot of energy instead of just a little energy into your projects and desires.

Your angel guidance is to create a wave of action. If you are unsure what step to take next, ask your angels and then listen and/or pay attention to the signs we put before you, for there are many indeed. We speak to you through your thoughts and inspiration, through music, and through the words of others. If you think to yourself, "I wonder if that's a sign", then for sure it is and take action.

You are flying high right now, which can threaten others. Don't descend or fall victim to a well meaning friend who is not really supportive. Sometimes those who love you are just afraid of being left behind; others might display actions because of their own feelings about their life. Trust in your guidance. Soon others will be inspired by the example that you have set and that encourages them to explore and expand their light. And this is the best way to be in service to others.

Affirmation: "I believe in myself and my ability to take action that is required to do anything I desire."

89

New beginnings

Embrace the new in your life. Sometimes one clings to the old as that are familiar and sometimes change can be frightening. Call upon us whenever you feel lonely or afraid when facing new situations, people or projects, as well as when you are shedding and releasing your old self. Be open to new approaches to life. Allow yourself to be stretched and know that humans learn about themselves through change and new experiences.

Have faith that something new is on the horizon. Hold positive thoughts for yourself and others as you go through doors of change. Support each other and make it your aim to have a sense of satisfaction from a job well done as you move on to the new that is coming your way, even if you can't see it yet, just as the flowers bloom each year, so too shall you bloom once again.

Affirmation: "I embrace the new in my life as I release that which doesn't serve me or those around me."

90

Enjoy yourself

Take time each day for joy. Take time out to enjoy all the hard work you do every day. These moments bring you inspiration as it allows your mind to clear when you do something 'just for fun'. Enjoying yourself is just as important as having a meditation practice in your day. These two activities are vital to your wellbeing and enjoyment while doing your physical journey.

Your angel guidance is to go outside and play today (and everyday). Call up a friend, take a walk, go for a coffee, engage in some non-competitive sport, or perhaps see a movie that makes you laugh. Allow the activity to be a respite from your daily routine. These times of joy open up creativity and imagination and this helps to envision your desires, and happy outcomes.

Take time today to enjoy yourself, it truly is a beautiful day!

Affirmation: "I take time and space for myself to enjoy life."

91

You are powerful

The energy of heightened success is available now. You can manifest your thoughts and ideas right now, so choose them very carefully! Just as you are capable of manifesting masterpieces, you are also capable of manifesting problems and chaos. Angel wisdom reminds you that you are also able to undo any manifestations that you are unhappy with in your life.

Use the alchemy of spirit to turn ordinary events and projects into something extraordinary. You have the power to make these endeavours come alive with meaning and purpose. You have the power to bless and bring abundance to all that you desire to touch.

The gratitude and the joy that is felt in response to these beautiful creations are keys to amplifying your alchemical abilities. When you channel that energy, you become the Master.

Call upon your angels to assist you in enhancing any project you wish to undertake and transform, as it is our desire to be in the flow of service to humanity.

Affirmation: "I am powerful. I use my abilities to manifest my desires now. Thank you."

92

You are beautiful

Accept all aspects of yourself. Angel wisdom reminds you to see the beauty in yourself, see the beauty that is all around you and see the beauty in each other. As one begins to see the beauty they carry, it brings out the beauty in all those around you. Even the angry man on the corner has beauty; it just might be a little deeper and harder to find than in others.

True beauty comes from within one's own heart. Expect to see more beauty and it is amazing what you can notice around you, a kind word, gesture or action that truly stirs your love. There are many beautiful lights trying to shine all around. Take notice of them and more will occur.

Take a deep breath, close your eyes and ask your angels to open them to greater love and beauty. Then, open your eyes and see all the beauty that surrounds you.

Affirmation: "I am beautiful. I see beauty and love all around me."

93

Ideas and inspiration

Pay close attention to your new thoughts and ideas. The angels want you to notice and follow the ideas you have recently received. These thoughts are answers to your prayers for guidance, so don't discount them as mere imagination. The angels want you to trust in the messages and act on that trust. Have confidence in the messages and inspirations you receive for they are divinely guided when they come from that still, quiet place deep within. Act as if these thoughts are already manifested.

Use the energy of heightened success that is surrounding you right now. Watch your thoughts for there is a shorter time lag in your creations as you raise your vibrations. Your gratitude for your ability to manifest, and also the joy you feel in response to your creations are keys to amplifying your abilities to transform anything that you desire.

Affirmation: "I trust in the support of the Universe."

94

Surround yourself with positive energy

Surrounding yourself with positive people and situations that allow you to attract and create your intentions and future moments in their highest potential. Angel wisdom suggests that you use your skills and talents with intention. Eliminate power struggles, conflicts and competition, which come from an ego based desire to win. This promotes harmony and joy around you and a magical sense that all things are possible. Appreciate the gifts within each moment as this will allow you to attract and create all that you desire.

Avoid negative people, situations, and influences as much as possible. Avoid negative discussions with yourself and others, turn off programs with negative themes, and stay away from violent movies etc. This will assist you in cleansing any hidden blocks that could slow you down from manifesting the results you desire.

Affirmation:"I am surrounding by loving thoughts about myself and others, I am light."

95

Hope

Do not worry. Things will really be all right. The angels wish to remind you that the Universe wants you to have your heart's desires. It is simply waiting for you to believe you deserve it. It truly is a kind Universe and everyone within it is working in your favour, even if it doesn't always feel that way. There are really no tests, blocks or obstacles in your way, except your own projections of fear and failure into your future.

Take a moment and quiet your mind. Feel your angels caress as they encircle you with new energy of trust, hope, and optimism, and let these energies fuel your today's and tomorrow's. Ask your angels for help and they will fan the sparks of potential and bring them to life all around you.

Affirmation:"I hold positive thoughts and intentions for my todays and tomorrows and know that all of my expectations are fulfilled."

96

Forgive

We place people and situations on our path for opportunities to heal, grow and release. The angels are guiding us to release any negative patterns associated with past situations that can hold us back when we harbour unforgiveness within our hearts. Forgiveness doesn't mean you condone the behaviour of another, it means that you are no longer willing to carry around the toxic thoughts and feelings within yourself. If you hold these thoughts within you, they will eventually appear as physical manifestations of illness, fatigue, depression, etc.

Begin by breathing deeply, releasing all negative thought patterns with each exhalation, giving your fears, worries, anger, and any painful emotions to the angels. See the Divine light and goodness within yourself, and then see this spark which resides within everyone. Encircle yourself and others in the Divine love of the creator, and watch as the energy around you transforms.

Focus upon your desires instead of fears or judgment. Release, be free and experience positive patterns that emerge from these hidden blessings.

Affirmation: "I choose to hold only loving thoughts in my heart and mind."

97

Work your magic

You are a magical Being. Now is the time to manifest your dreams and desires. You are a powerful creator, the challenge is in remembering where your thoughts are and to keep your focus on that which you want, not what you fear.

Tap into your magical abilities which you have used successfully in the past. Pull these abilities out of storage and use them to work magic now. Your clear and focused intentions, positive expectations, prayers, affirmations, and action steps all create the healings and manifestations you desire. So work your magic each day.

Affirmation:"I am powerful. I have the power to create magic in my life."

98

You have a gift

Each of you is a unique gift. Each of you has your dance, that is uniquely yours and no one else will bring that energy to the earth journey with quite the same pizzazz that you bring with you.

We offer you our love and support and that you may also feel the love and support that you currently have in physicality with you.

Celebrate the gift that is you, just as we did when you decided to come to the Earth realm. Feel the heart open and expand as you wear the true mask that is you. Dance your dance, sing your song and do it from love. We are truly grateful to share in your journey. Be joyful in your opportunity to do the dance.

Affirmation: "I dance to the rhythm of life. My life is a celebration and I offer myself to be in tune to that dance."

99

Discipline

It is time to release old patterns. Release old memories, ingrained habits and mental patterns which lower you vibration. With order and some discipline, your life runs more smoothly. This helps to bring you more clarity and joy. It helps keep your focus and keep things moving.

You are reminded that you are a beautiful, light, and wise spirit and that only the material mantel disguises the spirit that you really are. So envision yourself surrounded by pure white light. Let your perfect spirit emerge and fly.

Use affirmations each morning as this will assist to open the flood gates of manifestation and help you keep on task with what you want to create. Be open to giving and receiving love. Reignite the passions in your life.

Affirmation: "Creating order and discipline helps me in creating the life I want for myself. I am pure and light."

100

Emotions

Let your emotions heal. This enables you to open yourself and your heart to greater love. Ask your angels to help you dissolve any feelings of anger, resentment, regret, unforgiveness, worry, sorrow and any other emotion that needs to be transition into another state of energy. See the gift that lives within each experience for it is always there. Ask your angels to help you transition any energy that no longer serve the growth of your soul.

Release and transformation is sometimes difficult to start, however the end rewards are worth the effort and journey. Remember to journal your progress as it will help to show you how far you have come when you stop to pause along the way.

We put many signs upon your path to help to guide the way. Notice them, for they are there. And as you do, more will become evident. This adds an almost magical element to your experience, so expect them, look for them and yet also detach from how they arrive, let it be that you know they are from spirit and enjoy the experience.

Affirmation: "As I heal my heart, more love comes my way."

101

Health and healing

Healing is a natural part of being and your healing thoughts are manifesting into physical form. Sometimes a situation can't be healed until the challenge is completely released, so that healing light can enter.

If you have been feeling stuck or indecisive, listen to your intuition about the circumstances surrounding you and then make the decision to move forward. To realized this healing, first stop focusing on 'what went wrong' and instead focus on what you have learned in the process, what you did right and what you will do differently in the future.

Hold thoughts of love around any situation that needs healing in your life. Angel wisdom reminds you that when you aim for a vision without doubt or deviation, it will succeed. Your guidance is to persevere towards your vision. Let every thought, word and action be directed towards your desired outcome.

Affirmation:"Everything is in Divine and perfect order right now."

102

Strengths

Focus on your Strengths. Release any thoughts of weakness and focus upon your strengths. By having your mindset on that which is more desirable, you will attract more of the same. You truly have no weaknesses, and you can't do things wrong. Everything is alright. You are alright.

Your strengths could include your loving heart, pure intentions, people skills, hobbies, or anything you excel at. You are always growing and improving. That which you focus on is what you create, so please spend as much of your day as possible focusing and improving that which ignites passion in your heart. Focus on what brings you closer to your Divine purpose.

Use positive affirmations daily to lift your energy and keep your spirits high. Speak of yourself and others in positive terms. Begin a physical exercise program that strengthens you. We bring you this message of love and healing. We are with you, giving you strength and courage to make life changes that will help work on your Divine life purpose.

Affirmation: "I face my day with strength and wisdom."

103

Serenity

Find the contentment. Regardless of where you find yourself, find peace in that moment. Take action based on your truth, and trust your inner guidance, and lovingly assert yourself by speaking with your heart.

Your angel guidance is to find your still, quiet center, then heal any anger, purify your emotions and trust your own judgment, and make your decisions from this point of your inner Divineness. True strength is based on inner strength, self worth and confidence. It is time to claim your birthright and be that powerful light that you are.

Affirmation: "I am serene, powerful and confident. I speak my truth from my heart."

104

New beginnings

Let the new of the world inspire you. Everything happens in cycles, and new life is making its way for half of your planet and going to sleep on the other half, and after its slumber, it will awaken to the new again. Take some time and listen to the birds, listen to the trees, listen to the grass. It is so beautiful to feel that energy, to touch it, to taste it.

Your angel guidance is to spend some time out of doors, breathing in the life that is around you. Allow it to penetrate your senses. Open your windows and doors and let in the finest molecules of the oxygen. And, savour each moment. Enjoy the sensations that are all around you.

Affirmation: "I experience more aliveness as I embrace the new all around me."

105

Synchronicity

Each event in your life is carefully orchestrated, by you, your guides and angels, so recognize them as the hand of spirit. As you start to expect them to occur, you will notice them more and know that they are a validation that you are on the best possible path at this time. Angel wisdom reminds you that the path your on is not set in stone, there are lots of alternatives and opportunities to change and shift what road you are taking. Awaken to the unlimited possibilities that are before you always.

Be at peace with yourself and where you are at. Remember that divine timing means that all things happen when each one is ready and that it is for the good of all. Being at peace brings you a new tranquility and a smoother road ahead. Trust and enjoy the beauty of now.

Affirmation: "I notice and appreciate the signs that let me know I am exactly where I need to be at this time."

106

Spiritual practice

Now is the perfect time to create a spiritual practice.

Your angel guidance is to create a daily spiritual practice for yourself. Set aside time each day to be alone and meditate upon what you truly desire. Visualize it, and it will come about.

Negativity will block your progress, so avoid negative situations, people and transform your thoughts. Any thought that is less than supportive and love should be transformed into a positive one that sees your desires happening now before your eyes.

Also spend some time each day doing an activity of playing and having fun, if possible, go outside. Take a walk, play a non-competitive game, or go visit a nature center or botanical garden, play on a swing. Playing creates joy and joy creates miracles and manifestation.

Affirmation: "I ask for and receive assistance to find and follow my higher path."

107

Go for it

Take action today. Your prayers and positive expectations have been heard and are being answered. You have indeed tapped into the unlimited supply of Divine guidance. As you invoke your angels, we begin to work behind the scenes, setting up situations and people to assist you along your path.

It is important that if you are asking and think that you are not receiving, that you quiet yourself and listen for the Divine promptings within you. Take steps today that lead you closer to that which you desire. Even if they are baby steps, you will feel lighter and brighter as you move closer to your goals. As you notice the magic around you, you begin to create more of it in your life. You are indeed a powerful creator and together we can go far indeed.

Affirmation: "Each day I am at least one step closer to creating what I desire."

108

Playfulness and fun

Fun and play is the angel's way!

We are guiding you to add more fun to your life. The angels want you to know that adding fun can assist you in reaching your goals; it is a wonderful investment that reaps great rewards.

When you laugh, you relax. This place of relaxation gives you a greater flow of ideas, spiritual connections, divine guidance, and energy. With new inspirations and energy, you are better able to manifest that which you desire. Your relaxed, radiant personality attracts new and helpful people and situations to you. You become more positive and then attract more wanted opportunities.

Go out and have some fun today!

Affirmation: "I find now things to be grateful for each day."

109

Focus on service

Now is the time to learn. Now is the time to gather information. If you are unsure what direction to take and feel you are not being guided, take some time to just be in the moment and serve humanity in some way that brings you joy. Put your entire focus on "how may I serve," and it puts you in a joyous stream of bliss that continually feeds you everything that you need. Be patient with yourself and do something that you love that also helps others along the way.

It is so much easier to attract that which you desire in your life when you are in this stream. So, keep charging ahead and come from that place of love and inner joy. As you stay in this energy, it affects everyone and everything around you.

Affirmation: "I joyfully serve humanity, for myself as well as others."

110

Take good care of yourself

When you make taking care of yourself a priority, everyone benefits. Your angel guidance is to give yourself something special today. Perhaps a relaxing treat like a massage, a sea-salt bath, a manicure or pedicure, or perhaps both. Do something that is new for you that you have always wanted to do for yourself. Make yourself feel special in some way, as each of you is very special indeed.

When you feel good about yourself, it is so much easier to open yourself up to unconditional love. Close your eyes, focus your breath, then your heart and let love flow from you and touch those you love, those you don't know and also those you are not particularly fond of at this time. This assists in creating the rainbow bridge of light which we angels can more easily move along to bring hope, love and peace.

Affirmation: "By taking care of me I have more to give to others. My heart is filled with love for all things."

111

Change in direction

When you come to a fork on your path, take a moment, focus on your breath, place your hand on your heart chakra and ask, "Which way brings me closer to my Divine purpose? Which way takes me away from it?" And, from that still, quiet space listen carefully for the prompting of spirit.

The changes that you are experiencing are divinely directed by your willingness to open your heart to love and to your inner guidance. Trust that you are always protected and can clearly see where the path before you will lead you. This is all part of your spiritual growth.

Angel wisdom reminds you that there is truly no wrong path to take, for each one leads you to an awakening that assists in your desire of evolution.

Affirmation: "I am always in the right place at the right time and notice the signs that are put before me."

112

Enjoying the moment

Remember a moment that touched your heart. Feel that love now and let that love envelop you, and flow over you. Just let the feeling flow and sit in that energy for awhile. Perhaps try this exercise in a garden, in the forest, by the ocean, or overlooking a view that you absolutely love. And, from this moment and energy begin to create.

Use this memory to fuel your passions. Use it to visualize your desires. Use it to spread love to others, especially those in need. Send that love in your Smile, in your eyes and from your heart as you greet another today, and know we walk beside you, supporting you, loving you.

Affirmation: "I easily remember loving moments and thoughts and use them to assist me each day."

113

Appreciation

Send love to your beautiful Earth. This beautiful planet assists you in experiencing a human journey. Take some time out today and everyday to touch and love your beautiful Mother Earth. She gives you each everything you need to sustain physical life and surrounds you with love and beauty always.

Your angel guidance is to quiet yourself and feel the love that she shares with each of you. Spend time feeling the trees, the plants and the waters. Share your love with her, for she is always a grateful recipient.

Affirmation: "I love and appreciate this beautiful earth that supports my life."

114

Truth seeker

Look for the real meaning of life, and see the two sides of the world. As you explore your spirit self and how to work with that part of you, also look for the meaning of your physical experience and how to blend these two aspects of you together.

Your angel guidance is to spend time in the physical world during your spiritual pursuits. Meditate and work with your guides and angels cradled in the beautiful bosom of Mother Earth. This allows for a rising in your vibration to bring us closer together. We are your teachers, your companions, your guides and together we form a circle that creates a harmonious whole.

Have faith that your prayers are manifesting. Remain positive, especially in the times when you feel you are alone, as these are the opportunities to connect with us and gain your clarity and direction. We are always with you, available for support and divine guidance. Just call and we will make ourselves known to you, watch for the signs, and recognize them as the hand of spirit.

Affirmation:"I see the truth in all things. I am surrounded by love and support always."

115

Purpose in life

If you are feeling unsure of what your purpose is, focus on something that makes your heart sing.

Your angel guidance is to find a project or hobby, or volunteer in an area that feeds your soul. This is the fastest track to finding your life purpose in that moment. As you discover a purpose, your purpose can change, so don't feel like you have failed or were wrong about the direction that you took. It is that you are now different and have something different to offer the world.

Look for the signs and synchronicities, as these are orchestrated by your guides and angels. Your angels speak to you through your dreams as well, therefore we encourage you to keep a dream journal and look for the similar theme or realization.

Angel wisdom reminds you that your prayers and questions are being answered. Notice them in order to increase their flow.

Affirmation:"My purpose is changing as I master one area

and move on to another. All things happen in perfect timing."

116

Sensitivity

You may find you are extra sensitive right now. You are becoming more sensitive to the energies and the emotions that are around you. Honour yourself, honour your feelings. As you awareness becomes greater, you become more sensitive to the thoughts and feelings that are around you.

Avoid situations that over stimulate you as you become acclimatized to this new way of experiencing the world. As you may find food or household products such as cleaners and soaps need to be changed to more natural, healthful products. Also, shed what you do not need and make way for the new to enter. Pay close attention to the loving guidance you hear inside of your mind and from other people as well. If it registers with you, follow it.

Give your cares and your worries to us angels, and us to take your burdens. We can assist in their transformations, invite us in, we are always here by your side.

Affirmation: "As I become more sensitive, I see, sense and feel the world in a heightened way."

117

Focus

Keep your focus on your highest priorities. We will help you get organized and motivated. We are your assistants and we will gladly help you get rid of clutter, and clear the energy around you. Clearing your environment enlivens the energy that surrounds you and therefore that which you attract to you.

Your angel guidance is to also clear the energy within you by clearing and opening your chakras. We will use sacred geometric shapes to assist in this process as well as in adjusting your programming for the new you that is always being created. You are evolving and shifting your vibration on many levels, dear ones. Be gentle with yourself as the process emerges. And in the light of the beautiful you that others can then see, they will ask you how you got so bright. It is then that you share with them your process of love.

Affirmation: "I focus my attention on my highest priorities."

118

Healing thoughts

As you reflect on the past, be sure to see the wisdom within the lesson. And, then release it and move forward. Sometimes things can't be healed until you release the challenges in your lives, so that then the healing rays can enter. Stop focusing upon "what went wrong" and instead focus on 'what you did that was right.' It is okay to trust that you are on the right path and then decide that it isn't working for you and make a course adjustment. Everyone and everything is put on your path for a purpose, even if you can't see that at this moment.

Your angel guidance is to infuse loving thoughts into all aspects of your life. This is the greatest healing you can give yourself. There is no such thing as missed opportunities, for if you had gone a different way, you wouldn't be the magnificent light you are now, or the one you are becoming with each decision that you make.

Affirmation:"Everything is in Divine and perfect order right now!"

119

Changing relationships

As you change, so too do your relationships with others. Now is the time to release any unfulfilled expectations from the past. It is time to open your heart to the greater and deeper love that is the natural flow as you release in order to expand. As you expand your heart, all of your relationships change. Some will drift away; others will find new heights and depths.

Your angel guidance is to look within your heart and really look deep. Ask your inner child what thoughts of love it is holding within. Oftentimes humans hold unrealistic expectations of love made from that place of protection of the child. Look within and ask yourself though meditation. Ask for angel guidance and support if you are unsure how to do this. We are always, always here to assist your journey.

Affirmation:"I am whole and complete within myself."

120

Spiritual practice

It is an important time on your journey to take care of yourself, not only physically, but also emotionally, mentally, and spiritually. Now is the time to focus on you. This is not to say, be selfish, but put yourself first. When you are in a state of balance, harmony and joy, you are of far better service to the Universe and those you love. It is time to focus with purposeful action and intention on where you need to have balance in your four realms.

Check within your inner beingness to see if you are out of balance in any of these realms and ask us to come and assist you in finding creative and fun ways we can bring that balance back. The very process of checking in each day is a huge part of balancing the spiritual realm.

Spend time each day in nature, or create your own little sanctuary of plants and flowers, and commune with Mother Earth, connect with your physical world, and eat live foods from the earth, swim and play in her waters. Read books, take classes, listen to and immerse yourself in activities that help you grow and evolve, that nourish your soul. Meditate, meditate, and meditate.

Let your heart expand; do the work of surrendering and releasing unfulfilled expectations and thoughts of unforgiveness. See the gift and the beauty in all things and move forward with your truth, trust and passion.

Know that this is not always easy, especially in the beginning of expansion, yet as you move forward, you will see the lightening on the path and will feel the joy and the peace you have been longing to create in your life.

WE are always here to assist you. ASK and we are there, whether you can feel us yet or not, we are there. Trust in what you feel in your heart.

Affirmation: "I am free of out dated, limiting beliefs. I see love and beauty all around me."

121

Hope

Keep hope alive in your heart. As you do you will feel the sun is about to come out in an area of your life. Your angels wish to remind you that your spirit recovers quickly when you keep faith with your dreams and visions. Remember the Universe wants you to have your heart's desire. It is simply waiting for you to believe you deserve it. Look at what thoughts might be holding you back or blocking the progress you desire.

Do your part by deciding what you truly want. Ask yourself, "What can I do to bring this into my life now?" and then, send out positive thoughts for the changes you seek and for the fulfillment of your dreams.

When you believe in positive outcomes, you attract the great and beautiful experiences into your life.

Affirmation:"I know I can do it. I am eternally optimistic."

122

Pay attention

Notice repetitious signs and your inner guidance, as this can yield valuable information. Rejoice when you notice them and more will come. These are your angel's messages, the answers to your prayers.

We are sending you wonderful ideas and wisdom, and these are very real and trustworthy. Spend time working with your guardian angels for they are simply here to support you throughout this incarnation. They have nothing but omnipresent love for you and desire to be of service.

So ask them for the signs to be put before you, ask them to surprise you with them, and you will know that they are a sign from them.

Affirmation: "I recognize the hands of spirit helping to guide my life."

123

Discovery and change

If the quest for balance and harmony is challenging you at this time, it is because change is inevitable. You may feel a little out of control with all the change that is happening around you, but you do have the freedom over how you choose to respond to change. What seems calamitous in the present moment may truly be your greatest opportunity for growth and change. Life is simply taking you on a ride right now and while you need to go on this ride, you don't need to scream with fear. Through this you will discover many things about yourself, but then, isn't this is what all truly great adventurers do.

Angel wisdom reminds you to find that calm, steady approach to understanding the components that will help you bring that balance and harmony back into your life. If you think creatively, and then use a well thought out process, you can bring seemingly opposing elements into harmony. There is a way to fuse your life, with creativity, clarity and intention, and then begin to work from that perspective.

Affirmation: "I am eager to explore and discover what life has to offer. I am in balance with my higher self and what I want to accomplish at this time."

124

Understanding

Seek understanding and wisdom within yourself and your experiences. Your angel guidance is to examine yourself and your current situations in depth so that you have a crystal clear awareness of the underlying reasons for any challenges and repeated scenarios.

Self-awareness is the foundation on which we build strong and healthy relationships, friendships and life experience. Understanding your thoughts, ideas, emotions and beliefs is a basis for understanding your spiritual self and your mission for doing the earth journey.

Spend some time contemplating the gift that is you. Look at the aspects of your personality and your responses to events, situations and people; see them with love (not self judgment) as the angels see you. Ask us for assistance to open your heart. Converse with us as we can help you to find your clarity and solutions that can assist you in having a more joy filled journey.

Affirmation: "I allow each and every moment to unfold with perfection. I seek to understand and transform any challenges in my life."

125

Supported and loved

You are not alone and you are safe. Each person is surrounded by a team of angels and ascended masters who are honoured to help you and want to offer guidance and always give you their love and support. Have mental conversations with them about anything and everything, and as you do you begin to see more evidence of their existence, and experience more of the gifts and guidance they offer humanity. If you ever feel doubtful, ask the angels to help you release these fears.

Your angels see only love within all that you do, and we ask that you learn to see the love within yourself and those around you. Ask us for guidance and trust your intuition. As you develop and use your intuition and trust, you feel safer, happier, stronger and clearer.

Affirmation: "I am empowered and enlightened by my inner guidance and my angels."

126

Serenity

Choose peace and tranquility. Peace of mind means feeling secure, and knowing that you've always provided for. Even if the logical mind cannot fathom how a challenge could be resolve, peace of mind means that you trust that your angels, guides and the Creator will assist you in creating miraculous solutions. This sort of trust is always warranted because faith is a key component in experiencing miracles.

The angels wish to reassure you that peace of mind is within you, it comes from within you. You can feel serene, even in the midst of great turmoil. Please don't think that you have to wait until your life is problem free before you can be happy and peaceful. The opposite is actually true. First, you work toward serenity, and they your life challenges lessen and disappear. Serenity is your natural state of being, and the angels are now working with you to actualize this.

Affirmation: "I choose to be happy now. I believe in myself."

127

Be joy filled

When we are connected with each other's light, there is much Joy. Together we are illuminated. When you remember that connection at any time, you are once again illuminated. And, as you stay in that place of light, you become a guide for others to see. Seek the light in the heart of each person you greet. Delight in all that is around you. Enjoy life.

Take time out to connect and bring that light into your aura. As you do this it affects those around you and they begin to seek brightness in their lives and it lights the way for the shift in consciousness that is happening on earth at this time.

Affirmation: "I connect with my light and merge it with the angels. I feel the joy in all that I see."

128

Unconditional love

Love yourself, others, and every situation. No matter what the outward appearance may be. To help to heal any situation or relationship, see the other person's point of view with compassion. Instead of seeing someone or something as 'good' or 'bad', have compassion, and know that everyone is doing the best they can at the time. Instead of pitying someone, see that person's inner strength and Godliness. This encourages the Divine light to be expressed within the other person as well as yourself.

There is a solution to every problem, so look at all things with eyes of love. Focus your thoughts on the beautiful things that you can find in people or situations and raise your light above all appearances, and see only love.

Affirmation: "I am one with the Divine, just as everyone and everything, and it is here that I choose to reside."

129

Empowerment

You are a powerful being of light. Use your powers with compassion and love. The angels wish to remind you that you are made of magical, omnipresent, creator energy. It is inside of your every cell. As you go and transform how you see and view your world, you become even more powerful, with more abilities. It is safe for you to use your powers, as you have learned of compassion and are learning the power of the light.

Each day take some time to increase your light, encircle yourself in a cocoon of light and love from your angels before you begin the day and at any time you feel you need to increase your light.

It is time to take your place as the powerful being that you are.

Affirmation:"I am powerful; it is safe for me to use my abilities to make a better world for all."

130

Answered prayers

Accept your angels help, for we are indeed surrounding you, supporting you, and lighting the way. Take a moment, take a breath, and look at the path before you. It takes conscious effort on your behalf when you first start looking for the signs that are answers to your prayers.

Reward yourself for a job well done, always. For you cannot do it wrong. There is no such thing as failure in this great universe. This is your mental body's response from the ego. It is truly offered in love to you as a form of self protection. It is time to love that part of you who thinks it keeps you safe, and give it a new program to follow as your guardian at the gate.

Affirmation: "I am free of outdated and limiting beliefs."

131

Lightworker

You are a Lightworker. Shine your Divine light and your love. Beam it from within you, and it lights the way for others. Let them come to you when they are ready. Until then, just keep shinning your light in the darkest of places. It is not always an easy path for the Lightworker, however, when you get to the point in your evolution it won't seem like same work you started.

Be open and flexible along the way. Ask your angels to help you open your mind and your heart with new ideas and fresh options. When you accept the possibility that there are other ways, previous unseen doorways will be opened to you and you can easily move through any change.

See the world through the eyes of your angels, with love and acceptance of all things, regardless as to how they appear at the present time.

Affirmation: "I am free to choose, I am flexible."

132

Hope

What do you desire right now? Visualize it, and it will come about. Stay positive, and know that you are a powerful creator. Any thoughts that are less than you desire, will bring results that are less than. Believe in yourself, believe that you are worthy and that all you desire can and will be yours. Be ready to receive it into your life. Do your part by deciding what you truly want. Send positive thoughts for the changes that you seek and for the fulfillment of your dreams.

Ask your angels for help and they will fan the sparks of potential and bring them to life.

Affirmation: "I am worthy. I am optimistic. I am ready to receive good in my life."

133

Honesty

What vibration are you holding? Your every thought, word, emotion, and action is reflected in your aura. When you are honest, your aura is crystal clear. Angel wisdom reminds you to radiate a resonance of honesty. When you are totally honest with yourself, you act with integrity and dare to be open, for there is nothing to hide. You create a vibration of respect and trust.

Keep charging ahead. Expect miraculous solutions to appear before you on your path, and they will. Look for the doors that are open for you now, and trust that more will be available to you. Trust that there is indeed enough for everyone.

Affirmation: "I am honest in my thought, word and deed. Miraculous solutions appear before me and I know what my next best step to take is."

134

Choose again

You have the freedom to choose again. Sometimes you feel tied down to a situation or person because they feel safe or we are honouring an obligation. However these circumstances can lead to being untrue to your authentic self and are acting the way you feel you should in order to keep the status-quo. To be free, you must rediscover your authentic self and walk away from that which no longer serves you or the good of all.

The angels ask you to realize that you are free. Living in freedom is simply a shift of mindset or attitude. Do not be afraid to let go of the familiar, for the new cannot come in until the old and worn out has been released. Transformation is a vulnerable time, so take care of yourself as you change.

Everything you do in your life is by choice, and you are free to choose again. The next time you begin to think "I have to", stop and explore new ways of thinking, doing, and being. Explore and experiment with new thoughts and ideas. Ask your angels to help guide you to complete tasks with a new attitude so you don't feel trapped or we can guide you to do something completely new in a way that brings you the freedom and joy you desire.

Affirmation:"I welcome new adventures and opportunities into my life."

135

Celebrate your progress

Today is about celebrating who you are and how far you have come. Take some time to celebrate who you are and the transformations and expansions you have made on your journey. It isn't always an easy task to be in a human process, yet the joy, rewards, and expansion that you have experienced as a soul has been astounding.

Look into your heart and see that you have come through many tests and trials and there were many times you felt you might not make it out of the forest, feeling there are so many obstacles, that it just isn't worth the journey. Yet at other times you have created magnificently, and felt so much love and joy. Lean upon us if you need courage and strength. Trust that you have indeed made tremendous progress and that each day is better than the one before.

Your angel guidance is to celebrate today, and celebrate all that you have and do. Focus on the joy of today and trust that you can tackle tomorrow in a new light.

Affirmation:"I am joy filled, and love to explore the wonders of life."

136

It is time to move on

It is time to let go of the old, forgive yourself, and move forward. If you feel like your energy has been fragmented, it is time for adjustments. It is time to make room for new projects by letting go of the old first. Let go emotionally and intellectually. In other words, 'quit" or say 'good-bye" in your thoughts and in your heart.

Angel wisdom reminds you that everyone feels they have made a mistake now and then and it is normal to feel regret occasionally. Focus on your positive attributes, the lessons you've learned and release the rest.

Your angel guidance is to sit quietly so that you can find the stillness within. Then you can shine a pure, clear light into every area of your life. In the clarity of that light the angels will reveal a new way of being and doing. You will see things differently and be able to move forward with strength and clarity.

Affirmation:"I ask that all effects of past actions and decisions that are no longer important be undone in all directions of time and space, and I now release any guilt completely. I am worthy."

137

Stay optimistic

Your dreams are coming true. Angel wisdom suggests that you use your skills for the common good of all. Eliminate any power struggles, conflicts and competition and please don't quit right before the miracles begin to appear in your life. As you follow and honour your dreams, and follow the guidance of your heart, prosperity is coming your way. Don't let doubt block your progress.

Pay attention to the words you hear and the feelings you feel. Pay attention to the signs we put before you. If you are unclear where or what to do next, close your eyes, quiet your mind and place your hand upon your heart, when you have reached that still, quiet center, and feel the love of us flow out of your heart, ask your questions, and pause between them to hear answers, receive feelings or a knowingness. Then take the action you feel will bring you closer to that which you desire.

Affirmation: "I am in alignment with spirit and my higher self."

138

Assistance

Ask for assistance when you need help. We must be asked first to assist in the lives of our human charges. As soon as we are asked we immediately go to work on your behalf. Even if you don't see the results yet, we are busy setting up encounters with other human angels. Pay close attention to any repetitive signs to let you know that we are here and helping. Then, take the steps that feel right in your heart.

Choose to do that which fulfills you the most. To feel surrounded by love, open your heart to others. See only love and the divinity within each person you encounter, regardless as to how they appear. Draw from the limitless pool according to your belief in how much you deserve. Angel wisdom reminds you to believe in yourself and trust that all your desires will come to you on angel wings and that you deserve more.

Affirmation: "I deserve love, prosperity and success in all my endeavours, and so it is."

139

Transformation

Many of you are experiencing enormous change. Although it doesn't always feel pleasant at the time, the changes bring you great blessings and are truly answers to your prayers. Change means that you are evolving as you should be. Ride the flow with the focused intention of opening yourself up to whatever is before you. For now is the perfect time to act upon your inspirations.

Use your favourite affirmations, and keep them with you during this time of transformation. These will help you keep your focus on creating what you desire. Angel wisdom reminds you that everyone and everything are on your side, supporting you always. If the current path you are on seems particularly arduous, know that you are being asked to release something that no longer serves you. And, as this energy is released, a beautiful new you will emerge.

Affirmation: "I give thanks for shedding the old. I welcome the newness of the gifts that are bestowed upon me."

140

Own your power

Be the magical light that dwells within you. The angels wish to remind you that everyone and everything is made of omnipresent creator energy. Each of us has this light that dwells within that is connected to love and all that is. Your angel guidance is to let that light shine, and to consciously surround yourselves everyday in this light.

Take control and move forward with intention as this allows you to head in the direction in which you wish to go. Avoid negative people and situations that can draw you away from your path. Instead, stay focused on your dreams and move determinedly, with purposeful action towards that which you desire. Be the inspired warrior of light that you are.

Affirmation: "I am focused and moving forward. I am surrounded by wonderful blessings at all times."

141

Divine magic

Expect miracles! Angel wisdom reminds you that you are surrounded by magical energy all of the time, it is when you trust in and expect miracles to happen that they begin to occur more frequently for you. Tap in to this reservoir and enjoy the magic you create. Take time each morning to set your intent see miracles around you, big and small. Feel the joy in the faces of those who are affected by this beautiful energy that you share. Enjoy yourself. This attracts more of the great and beautiful into your life.

You are safe and spiritually protected and you have a sacred mission to share light and love with your fellow travelers. Your joyful heart and light-hearted laughter sets your power into motion. Share it graciously.

Affirmation: "Miracles surround my thoughts and actions. I am guided by the energy of love and light."

142

Love and compassion

Life is full of changes and surprises. Ask your angels to help you open your mind and your heart to new ideas and fresh options. To heal situations in your life, see the 'others' point of view with compassion. This does not mean that you agree with them, for that is not always important. It is important however to give others time and encouragement to say what is in their heart as well.

Have confidence in yourself and your abilities. If this isn't possible just yet, trust in your angels and your guides. Learn to trust your own inner wisdom, for it is Divine guidance indeed. There is a solution to every problem, so see things with the eyes of love and expectation. And lean upon us if your confidence wavers, and we will buoy your courage and your faith.

Affirmation: "I am filled with more love and compassion each day for myself and others."

143

Developing your senses

Meditation is the perfect way to more easily hear and receive our messages.

Come and take a journey with us to a magical land and tap into your inner wisdom and work on expanding your senses. Relax and open your mind to receiving, without directing your thoughts. Just notice the feelings, visions, or ideas that come your way. Call in your entourage of angels to assist you and then be open to the expansion that is taking place.

And then, in your 'awake' state, notice the loving guidance you hear inside your head, or from other people. Notice the feelings that you get and trust in them. If you are unsure, quiet your mind and breath, and ask your heart center to give you more information and then act on the information you receive. Ask your angels to open your third eye and practice using these tools in your everyday life.

Affirmation:"Each day my senses are expanding, opening and becoming more sensitive."

144

What is truly important

Be open to your gifts. Ask yourself, what is truly important for me to spend time and energy on?"

Your Angel guidance is to look at your relationships, work, home, family, and the world that is around you. We want to help you understand and heal any imbalances that are occurring in your life. As you heal and release any feelings and thoughts that no longer serve you, the more rapidly you manifest your desires.

Focus on your highest priorities. In your mind and heart, surround any people, situations and yourself in an orb of loving energy; trust that love is the heart of the matter. Be open to the gifts within each situation and person, and allow yourself to feel peace, love and harmony. Celebrate the moments within each moment, for everything is there for a reason, to enable you to grow and evolve. This is the reason you came to do the earth journey, to grow and evolve.

Spend time on projects and activities that make your heart sing. Make choices that honour you and your current life's mission. Share your gifts with others so they too can find that peace and harmony.

Affirmation: "I spend my time wisely on what matters the most to me."

145

Positive change

As you grow, your likes change. As you change, you sometimes outgrow people, situations and circumstances that are not evolving; everyone evolves at a different rate. What is important is that these situations are growing as well, although perhaps in a different direction than you are, however, they all signal spiritual growth. Some of these situations push you beyond your comfort zone and these are the ones that are truly a blessing, as that discomfort is where you often do the most growing.

Angel wisdom reminds you that the Universe stands behind you, beside you and is always ready to support you. As well you have human angels who are also standing ready. Remember to ask as well as look around and see who is there as your earthy assistance. Trust that there are those around you who can help and they will be there, as if on angel's wings. As you evolve beyond your current self, you help others to awaken their spiritual gifts and get in touch with their Divine life mission.

Affirmation: "I cherish change as it signals that I am evolving and expanding and becoming a bright light to help humanity."

146

Dream big

Let go of any small thoughts for yourself and others. See yourself succeeding in any endeavour that you choose to focus on. Imagine it as happening in the most grandest of fashion, even bigger, more elaborate that you can possibly imagine. And as you do this, remember the exhilarating feeling that you feel and carry that energy with you. Every time you think of that desire, or take a step towards it, invoke that feeling.

Send positive thoughts for the changes that you seek as well as the fulfillment of your wishes. Ask the angels for help and they will fan the sparks of potential and bring them to life. Let your angels work on the details while you focus on the joy of having it.

Be at peace regardless. Angel wisdom reminds you that you can hover in the eye of any hurricanes that may swirl around you right now. Through breath and intention, you can stay centered regardless of what's happening in your life. This inner foundation of peace has a very powerful healing effect. As this happens, your outer life begins to reflect your inner one. Be at peace to ensure a peaceful outcome.

Affirmation: "I am at peace; I bring a new tranquility to my life and to a smoother road ahead. I am eternally optimistic. I deserve a grander life."

147

Endings

Endings lead to new beginnings. Many of you are ending a cycle in your life. Call upon your angels to comfort you, and to also guide you to your next step. Endings can sometimes be difficult, so we wish to remind you that happiness awaits you as you release that which no longer serves your growth.

Your angel guidance is to nurture your relationship with yourself, and that every other relationship follows from there. To attract, heal, release, or balance a relationship, ask the angels and guides to assist you. As you feel more loving to yourself, feel safe and loved within, all things around you become balanced, and can bloom and grow.

Affirmation: "I lovingly release [anything you need or want to release]. I am whole, safe and loved at all times."

148

See only love

See the love in everything. If you are being challenged right now in a certain area of your life, envision what the end result will look like, and feel like, then hold that thought with all the love and beauty you can possibly imagine. Ask yourself "How will I feel when I create the life I desire?" and then take steps towards creating that in your life.

The angels want you to know, believe and trust that they are working with you always behind the scenes, when you ask for their help, even if you don't see the results yet. Ask that your knowingness, strength and courage be increased. Keep your personal energy fields and your thoughts clear and cleaned every day. And, most importantly, see the love and beauty in all things, especially in the steps you've taken already on your own journey.

Affirmation:"I honour the love and the beauty within me, and radiate that love into all that I do."

149

Knowingness

You are a magical person. You can manifest all that you desire with your clear intentions. Each of you has the ability to tap into the universal pool of abundance. It is when you trust with a deep inner knowingness that you will begin to create, as if by magic. Angel wisdom reminds you when you believe that you are worthy and deserving, it is then that you stand fully in your power.

If you are confused and indecisive, it is because you do not have enough information. We ask that you do the research and seek expert advice. This will help you make decisions for yourself that you trust. Ask your angels to guide you and be open to the signs and human angels that are put on your path.

Affirmation: "I trust my inner knowing, I notice the signs from guides and angels quickly and easily, and we are always connected to each other."

150

Manifestations

Your aspirations are always available. Now is the time to take all thoughts and desires, and transform into tangible form. This is the time to take real control of consciously creating in your life. If things have looked bleak, it's time to turn this energy around.

First look at where your thoughts are. Thoughts are transformed into tangible things; they begin with an idea, then the idea meets with a feeling. If the feeling is loving and nurturing, the idea and the feeling create the embryo of the manifestation.

Things are going to change, the question is, which direction are they changing to? Rethink what you're going to do at this time. Meditate, keep calm, and take what action you can. Take good care of your health. Start reading, take time out for yourself, and turn your face to the sun. Take a walk in the woods, enjoy your loved ones, your food, and care for your health. Life is complex, yet so simple.

Angel wisdom reminds you that your intention into this new stage is a most important step and the universe's abundance is open to you. There may be a new beginning of some kind, and new challenges and opportunities are defiantly on the horizon. You are about to start another phase in your karmic journey, a brilliant new phase of this grand adventure called YOUR LIFE is about to enfold, embrace it with passion.

Affirmation: "My life is growing better and better each day."

151

Live your truth

Speak your truth. Live your truth, be your truth. It matters not what others are thinking or doing, it only matters how you feel about thoughts, words and deeds. The angels suggest that you look within and purify any murky thoughts and feelings and be totally honest with yourself. There is nothing wrong with your thoughts and feelings, of you living your truth honestly. Let those thoughts and feelings come from your heart, tempered always with love, a love that is unconditional. Let others be their own truth as well. If your truths differ greatly, take that as a sign to release that situation and move on to relationships that have a spiritual basis.

Be open to giving and receiving love in your life that is of a spiritual basis. These don't have to be exactly the same, as long as all parties are growing and evolving. There are many paths up the mountain and love and respect each person who lives their truth honestly. Accept all things with love, regardless as to how they appear.

Affirmation: "I love and respect all with unconditional love. I am honest and truthful in my thought, word and deed."

152

Divine timing

Your desired outcome will occur. Have patience and trust that it will happen. Relax and work with resolute focus toward that which you desire. Call upon your angels and guides to assist you along the way. And if your confidence waivers, we are here to buoy your spirit. Walk through the doors that are open and learn from the ones that are closed. We walk beside you, lighting the way.

You are becoming more sensitive to the world around you. As you raise your vibration, you will find that you are more sensitive to harsh chemicals, environments, situations and relationships. The angels wish for you to understand that all is perfect and is as it should be. Enjoy where you are right now, and know that this too will change as you change.

Affirmation: "All things happen in Divine timing. As I become ready for the next step, it appears before me."

153

Letting go

It is time to let go. The sun rises and sets each new day. Release the thought that you are not sure where to go or what to do next. Take some time to recharge, reconnect, and rejuvenate yourself. See the beauty within each moment and remember that each sunset brings the dawn of a new day. Look deeper into each situation you are releasing and see the gift that has been offered to you. Talk positively to yourself. Love yourself. Focus on the good in your life and let that grow and bloom.

Always keep your channels of communication open. Be a bridge to the hearts and minds of others, so that they too can find the peace, balance and harmony that releasing that which no longer serves you can bring. You are entering a new time of hope and fulfillment, and others will feel empowered to do the same by your example.

Affirmation: "I release negativity, I believe in positive outcomes for everyone."

154

Inner wisdom

Honour and follow your heart. As you learn to trust your inner wisdom, that part of you that is connected to your guides, angels, and the creators light, much more is available to you. Temper everything through the wisdom of your heart connection and see the love and the lessons within each experience and then release them and move on. Let your past go and make room for the new to come in. Trust that you did the best you could at the time with what you had to work with and release them with love.

Follow the guidance of your heart, and all that now is available to you will come your way. Connect to that still, quiet center within you, and listen to the promptings of spirit and your infinite self. When you trust your own connections, you gain a new perspective, and dramas and fears become unimportant, and a new peace and joy are yours.

Affirmation: "I connect and trust my inner wisdom. I am connected with my higher self, and am guided with love."

155

Adventure

Life is an adventure. Be ready for the unexpected and make the most of all opportunities. Do things that are different and approach life with a sense of wonder and joy, like when you were a small child and everything seemed new and magnificent.

If the path ahead seems dark, and the thoughts of moving forward seem scary, do as you would if you were exploring a dark place, and ask your angels to light the way. Watch for the signs that help you decide where and how to go.

Now is the perfect moment to forge ahead as your dreams are just around corner. Explore the new that is before you with excitement and courage, with anticipation, expectancy and hope.

Affirmation: "I face the adventures before me with excitement and anticipation."

156

Blossoming

Just like the flowers in the spring. There is always a resting period between the cycles.

You are just getting started, so have patience with yourself. Don't give up, as the process is just that, a process. Your angel guidance is to stop and smell the flowers along the way, to count your blessings and see the gift in all things. Say thank you to the Universe for all the gifts that have been so generously give to everyone and offer gratitude to the ones that are yours.

Take good care of yourself, begin a Yoga or exercise program that enhances your feelings of well being, and bring you peace of mind and spiritual growth at this time. Allow your physical vessel to catch up to all the changes that are occurring in your blossoming growth. And honour yourself always.

Affirmation: "I am grateful for everything in my life. I easily see the gift in all things."

157

The wisdom of solitude

Take some time to withdraw from worldly matters for a time to reflect and know your true self again. Look to understand what karma has been sharing with you. Sometimes you need to take yourself away in order to understand the true significance of what needs to be released, so you can move forward refreshed and wiser than you were before this respite from the world.

If the ghosts of the past are resurfacing, welcome them, for they still have something to teach you. Anything you may have fled from, people you may have unresolved issues with, memories of situations you wish you hadn't experienced may well be coming up. You might bump into someone from the past, dream of your ancestors, and be thinking of old times. The lesson here is that life is a circle and the wheel is turning, so move on, you need to take stock and reach a new level of understanding about your own actions, those of others, and reach an emotional level of forgiveness that may have challenged you in the past.

It is time to grow wiser, and forgive others and most importantly, yourself, and then things will heal and be complete. Through this flurry of strange events, you will be stronger, you will move on and you will continue to grow.

Affirmation: "I take time to review my life and be sure to complete undesired cycles. This allows me to move forward without restrictions."

158

Simplify your life

Life is full of many changes. Your angel guidance is to open your heart and your mind to all the possibilities that are out there. Find the gift and the wisdom within you which enables you to aspire to the knowing that there is so much more to experience. Then, expand your comfort zone so that you can explore your dreams.

Release people, situations and circumstances that don't serve your growth or are your responsibility. Oftentimes humans take the responsibility of the world upon their shoulders and it is time to release that. You are responsible for yourself and how you experience, react and behave, and let others take their power by letting them be responsible for theirs. Practice the art of forgiveness as this is so important when releasing your burdens. Focus on simplifying your life, and let others do the same for themselves when they are ready.

Laugh more, play more and enjoy life. There is so much that is wonderful all around you. Focus on the beauty and wonder of the journey and simplify your life.

Affirmation: "I release my attachment to people and things; all that I need is readily available to me."

159

Empowerment

You are truly powerful. It is safe for you to stand in your power and express yourself from your truth. In past lifetimes you have felt unsafe to be in your power. Angel wisdom reminds you that you are indeed a powerful creator, so choose your decisions and thoughts carefully. Release and surrender thoughts of less than. Open your arms and release any challenges that you have held so close to your heart, for it is time. The changes you experience are gifts you have requested, so please change the thoughts so the floodgates of manifestation can be opened and allowing.

Change brings great blessings so please embrace it as proof that you are evolving beyond where you currently are. You are safe and protected now, and in the future, so follow your path to the happy outcomes you desire. Use the power of affirmations daily. Open your hands, arms, mind and heart to your angels love and assistance and take your rightful place as the powerful creator that you are.

Affirmation: "I am powerful. It is safe and rewarding for me to be powerful. I release and surrender all thoughts of less than for I am deserving and worthy of all that I desire."

160

Self acceptance

You are beautiful. See the love and kindness that is within you, and share you love it with others. Sometimes life can be overwhelming and it is forgotten that all things begin with how you view yourself. See yourself as the beautiful light that you are, as we see you. Not by the physical or the mental self, see yourself from the spiritual/emotional self and that reflection will be a beacon for others to see themselves in a new light.

Watch your thoughts, as these are reflected in your aura. It is important to only think about or focus on what you desire.

Be kind to yourself. Have reasonable expectations and give yourself some due praise. In order to nurture the qualities that are yours, cherish yourself. Worry not what others are doing or thinking, focus on what you are doing and thinking. Your rewards will be a sense of inner peace, warmth and love. See yourself as the beautiful child who is part of the creator. Love yourself as we love you.

Affirmation: "I am beautiful. My inner light shines for all to see and feel. I am love."

161

Explore your options

It is a good time to explore. There are other possibilities and paths to take on your journey. Now is a great time to explore and change anything you are not happy about. Regardless of where you currently are, there are options available to you that you may not have thought of yet. This is a good time to ask your angels for assistance, for we are always ready to support you and guide your way. We don't do the journey for you, we assist you in seeing the bigger picture as well as lighting your way. You are always loved and supported for everything that you do.

Be honest with yourself, look into your heart and follow your truth. Consult someone who can assist you if you aren't sure exactly how to begin. You are part of an awesome group of beings whose focus is entirely about supporting and loving you, both physical and non-physical. Now is the time to use the resources that are available to you.

Affirmation: "I am always safe and supported. I receive constant love, guidance and support, always and in all ways. I choose the best path for me wisely."

162

Healing of yesterdays

It is time to let go of past power struggles. As you gaze and reflect on the past, be sure that issues, especially ones that were based in power struggles of the ego have been healed and released. Know that today and tomorrow can look very different from yesterday. The challenge lies in letting go of yesterday and focusing your attention on this moment. Your personal power and strength increase and grow as you let go of past power struggles.

Your angel guidance is to know that you are safe and protected at all times. Use affirmations of what you desire, as these open the floodgates of manifestation power. Look for things and thoughts that feel good and you feel good about, and from this new state of being, watch how everything in your life will unfold to reflect this new vibration of you.

Affirmation:"I see this day as a positive new beginning."

163

Peace and tranquility

Take some time to be still. Relax, and enjoy the introspection in the solitude it often brings. Indulge in some much needed self care. Take some time out in your day to be alone with yourself and think only beautiful and wonderful thoughts. Dream of your next holiday; look at the beauty that surrounds you. Yes, the angels know that sometimes you can look around and see only the dark, and it is in those times that it is so important to find the light in every situation, scene or episode in your life.

Take a walk in the park, smell the flowers, smell the rain. Feel the beauty that surrounds you. Notice the people who share love, pass on the rest during this respite from the world.

Your angel guidance is to remind you that your essence is divine and that is also the essence of every living thing. See the divine that surrounds you.

Affirmation:"I am serene, powerful and peaceful."

164

Teaching and learning

Keep an open mind, and learn new ideas and develop your philosophies, then teach these to others by your example. Teaching and learning are linked in a perfect cycle, in which information comes to you when you need it. Share with others about the topics that awaken your passions when they are ready to hear it. This is best done by walking your talk and when others are ready they will ask you what it is that allows you to feel confident, peaceful, grounded, inspired, serene, happy, and joyful. "What is your gift at this moment?" and live it from your heart. Be open to the gifts others have to share with you, for together you are more powerful than as a single entity on a solitary path.

Angel wisdom reminds you that preaching to others of your way does not serve the spirit. It is about being who you are and opening your heart to the sparks of potential and bringing them to life.

One of the great masters of your time left you with the most powerful information and did so by example, "You must be the change you wish to see in the world." And, all change begins by the one stepping forward and changing their own life first and others see the possibilities this brings to the world and they begin to change themselves.

Affirmation: "I accelerate my growth by living in my higher purpose."

165

Take good care of yourself

The angels urge you to care for your physical body. You are asked to eat healthful foods, to exercise regularly, and to avoid toxins of any kind, mental, emotional, and spiritual, as these make raising your vibration more difficult. The physical body is the densest and therefore requires extra care at this time.

Your angels are asking you to pay attention to your physical body; after all, you are here to have a physical experience. Perhaps you resist this guidance, and the angels have repeatedly come to you about this topic. They remind you that the body is an instrument that, when well tuned, emanates greater harmony. Your spirit is like the music of a grand piano, and the angels ask you to maintain that piano.

Your angels know that if you follow this guidance, you will feel better. Your increased energy and happiness is your reward for following the angels' suggestions. They will help you find the time and motivation to exercise. The will also help you lose your cravings for unhealthy substances. And, the angels will help you enjoy the new found pleasures that come from purifying and maintaining your physical body.

Affirmation: "Every cell in my body vibrates with energy, health and love."

166

Spiritual growth

You have the opportunity to embark on great change. New growth, psychic and spiritual experiences change the way you look at the world and yourself. As you evolve, allow your spiritual gifts to open. Share these gifts with the world. Invoke your angels and know that you are protected at all times, from all harm. Relax and enjoy the ride.

Renew your passion for life itself. Embark on a journey of health and healing. And, regardless as to what you've told, every one of you can have a long, healthy life, if you so desire. This might be some work and difficult at first, however it is a journey well worth taking, and we are always by your side, assisting you on the way.

Affirmation: "I choose to do things that evolve, inspire and uplift myself and others."

167

New opportunities

Something new is being made available to you now. And it is up to you to take advantage at this time. Be alert, be aware and be prepared, as you are surrounded by this new energy of creation that you have been working towards. Look at the past with love and blessings, and then move forward and grasp the new energy that is flowing your way. To increase this energy, relax and open your mind to receiving the messages from your angels.

Day dream regularly and be open to receive without directing your thoughts. Just relax and notice any feelings, visions, or ideas as if you were watching a movie. Then, move forward with the ones that feed your soul, your mind, and your heart.

Know that your angels are with you and surround you with love always and bravely move forward in the direction of your dreams, we are always at your side lighting the way that offers you the best possible outcome, pay attention to the signs and your dreams at this time.

Affirmation: "The abundant wealth of the Universe flows through me now."

168

Outcomes

Your focused intentions will occur. Have patience and trust; don't try to force things to happen. Detach from your desires once you have made your decisions and trust that your angels will take care of the details.

Your responsibility is to: Ask for help from your guides and angels, and you all have an entourage of light beings in various forms and from various dimensions who have agreed to be your assistance from the other side.

The second is pay attention to your inner guidance. Connect with your own deep knowing and you will be guided each step of the way. We talk to you through the prompting of spirit. Remember, your inner guidance is connected to us. So wear your golden cloak of wisdom always.

Be sure that you are not blocking your manifestations with contradictory negative thoughts. Use affirmations to help you stay focused, strong, and positive. Sometimes situations that appear negative to you are your greatest opportunities to grow and expand. Remember to see only the love within your experiences and be brave and look at what your next step is with us by your side.

Affirmation: "I am living my higher purpose and I do what brings me joy and I love participating in."

169

Clear intentions

Be clear about your desires. Focus upon them with truth, trust and passion. Now is the perfect moment for you to act on your inspirations. The doors are open, while you walk through them with the angels at your side. Everyone and everything is on your side, supporting your desired outcome. Don't procrastinate, as all the ingredients are ripe for your success. Allow yourself to imagine that your desires are already manifested and experience the emotional and physical feelings of your manifested desired.

Your angel guidance is to welcome the new in your life. If you are unsure what is the next best step for you to take, consult an expert. Once that first step is taken towards your desires, the Universe then gives additional help. Seek wise counsel from someone who has expertise in this area, and benefit from their knowledge and experience. To attract the right expert to assist you, be it an earthy being or your angels and guides, set your intentions and ask that they be drawn to you. Be open to where that assistance may come from.

Affirmation: "A helpful knowledgeable, experienced and wise being with integrity is available to me now, and able to assist me in all dimensions of time and space, the past, the future, the present."

And then, be open to the signs, take notes, and give thanks. Then, enjoy the results of your creations.

170

Love and joy

See only love. Spend some quality time with those that you love. Focus on the love that you feel when you just be with them, with no other agenda than love. Or, do something that brings you absolute joy. Walk in the sunshine along a shoreline with your dog. Walk in the beauty and freshness of a spring rain, Play with your kitty cat. Paint a picture of your favourite memory. Feel the love and the joy that being with one you love brings into your life and hold those thoughts whenever you feel sad or lonely. Tap into those beautiful memories and utilize that energy to transform the energy around you at any time.

Anytime you feel sad or lonely, close your eyes and remember the moment of love and joy that you created this day. Allow it to completely envelop you and just be in that energy. Then open your eyes and see only the love and gift that is being offered to you.

Remember the feelings and joy of just being. All the rest is just stuff along the way. Focus on Love, this will heal all things.

Affirmation:"I see the beauty and love in all things."

171

Trust and add more balance to your life

Learn to trust your gut feelings and intuitions, and regularly balance your time between work, play, spirituality and your relationships.

Use common sense and discernment and never give your power to another. Instead trust in yourself and your connection to the Divine wisdom that is a part of who you are. Keep purifying your motivations so that they are completely about love and service to elevate the energy and your experiences even further. Look past the seeming errors, and misunderstandings, and see only love within each person, and situation.

Your angels ask you to add regular doses of meditation, exercise, and play to your day. This helps you grow and bring more joy into life. If you are feeling overwhelmed by all your responsibilities, ask your angels to help to lift the burdens, and delegate that which you don't really need to do to make extra time for yourself and your own growth. This helps you to function better for yourself and therefore those in your life.

Affirmation: "I stay balanced and in my center at all times."

172

Focused intention

Your desired outcomes will occur. Keep your unwavering thoughts, feelings, and actions on that which you desire and they cannot help but appear before you. Have patience and faith, yet don't try to force it, work toward it.

Your angel guidance is to examine carefully your level of trust and believe that you will indeed be taken care of and all things are yours for the asking. There is enough for everyone and the Universe has an abundant supply of everything. Stay positive. Know what your priorities are and take action accordingly. Release any thoughts of doubt, or less than. And, avoid all naysayers and sceptics.

Affirmation: "I trust in the abundant supply of the Universe. There is more than enough for me and everyone."

173

Restoring balance

Look for resolutions that are available to you now. It is the perfect time to bring balance, temperance and harmony back into your life.

Are you tired of juggling everything in your life? Or riding the proverbial roller coaster of emotions, thoughts or finances, or perhaps all three? The angels remind you that life's journey can be what you make it. If you see only negative things, you will feel that you have bleak prospects in your future. If you feel the world is cruel and punishing, you will encounter lots of opportunities to see misfortune and anger, if you feel love and joy; you will see people who are happy, successful and expanding.

There is plenty of energy around that assists in seeing what you are feeling or resonating it back to you. Where are your thoughts? What is the world mirroring back to you? Do you see love around you?

Angel wisdom reminds you that now is the time to work on making life changes in how you see the world. Focus on being more conscious about where your thoughts are and where you want them to be. Be open to new ways and ideas from others who emulate those ideals and walk the talk.

The quest for balance and harmony can be challenging. It requires a certain kind of calm, steady approach and an almost scientific formula to understand the components that will help you plan a way to balance and harmonize your life. If you think creatively, and then use a well thought out process, you can bring seemingly opposing elements into harmony, whether it is friends and family, or aspects of your own personality, or work life. There is a way to transform your life: if you can fuse creativity and organization, you'll create a wealth of opportunity and enjoyment in your life.

Utilize the magnetic quality of this energy!

Affirmation: "I stay balanced and in my center at all times."

174

Compassion

To help to heal any situation, View circumstances from everyone's point of you. This might take a little time and you may have to stretch yourself sometimes, however filling your heart with compassion and understanding for others, or the situations they find themselves in, either with you or others is a gift of healing you offer yourself. Release any feelings of judgement, or good or bad, and see the strength and godliness within everyone.

If you struggle with this, ask your angels to send you a message that will help you to understand. We can help you see the bigger picture of life and to explore it with love and adventure. Take things one step at a time and take time out for you in between everything else.

Affirmation: "I am releasing that part of me that is irritated when I think of you. I am filled with love and joy now."

175

Time out

You are a Lightworker. You hold a space and share a light that is so necessary on the beautiful earth at this time that no one else has to share. We ask you to hold your divine light and love as much as you can at this time. Also please remember to balance that with time-outs for yourself. You are often so busy helping others that you forget to take care of you. And while it is exceptionally important for those awakening to beam that love and light, you can't be of service to others if you don't take exceptional care of yourself first.

Plan regular sojourns in mother nature, run, play and enjoy that beauty that surrounds you, pamper yourself with a nice hot sea salt bath, a pedicure, a massage, and one of the best ways is to receive an energy healing session. Plan a healing share with some of your Lightworker friends or go to a healing workshop for yourself as well as to add to your medicine chest.

Please remember that you are a beautiful and valued member of a very important team and we want to assist you in any way we can, so please do call upon us for guidance and we will immediately go to work on your behalf. Ask to be open to receive.

Affirmation: "I create quiet time to seek the guidance and clarity that I need to assist in my growth."

176

Love life

Happiness and bliss are your birthright. And, they are a natural state of being. This is what life is all about. When you are in love with life itself, the rest of the world can feel your light and it assists others to awaken. This is how the world is changed, one person at a time finding happiness and bliss, regardless of the circumstances that are surrounding them.

This is not always an easy task as a human; however we say to you that it is this very step that will indeed move mountains.

What is truly important in your life? Is it the things that you have bought or acquired? Is it when you have loved and felt the love of someone else?

Your angel guidance is to keep your loved ones close to you, and hold each other. Hold your loved ones on a cold night; hearing your child say 'I love you'; watching your garden grow; watching a sunrise, watching a sunset, watch children play at the beach, what makes your heart sing? Love the very moment of life itself in all of its glory and glow with that love.

Affirmation: "I follow my bliss. I have what is important to me in my heart. I am surrounded by loving people."

177

Be free

Freely express your true self. You are a beautiful part of the creator and let no one diminish you. Realize you have the power to be free, and freedom will follow. Everything you do in life is by choice, whether or not that is clear to you. You are free to choose your thoughts, regardless of the circumstances that surround you. Ask your angels to help you find alternatives if you feel stuck and trust that it will come your way.

Make time in your day to do something that brings you absolute joy and allows you to just be in the moments of joy and freedom. This assists in creating energy for you to feel free from any restrictions that you might feel bound by, and in those moments your angels can offer you inspiration and help you temper all things with love. Practice yoga or some other form of movement, or make up your own and feel the freedom of breathing and moving to the rhythm of the Earth. This helps bringing you peace of mind and assists in your spiritual growth.

Affirmation: "I am always free to choose my thoughts and mind set."

178

Blessed change

Life changes bring you great blessings. The sun sets and rises each day, as it is with the adventures in your life. See the beauty within each sunset in your life, and know that the sun will also rise again tomorrow. Endings are merely the start of a new beginning. Tap into your connection with your inner divine guidance. This wealth of knowledge is available to each of you, should you choose to take the time to connect and solidify this connection.

The angels wish to remind you that gaining a clearer connection takes practice, as does your trusting in these connections and messages. Use affirmations daily to assist in keeping your focus positive as you go through the endings and start the new beginnings. These help to change where your thoughts are, and how to focus where your attention should be. The angels urge you to stay centered and focused in a state of grace and acceptance as you move forward, leaving behind that which no longer serves you.

Affirmation: "I welcome Divinely Inspired change, I am centered."

179

Speak your truth

Communicate what is in your heart. Share your truth by speaking from your heart. For as you communicate with others using your heart as the filter, others feel you're the resonance of your words and trust what you are saying. There are always ways to be truthful without hurting others feelings if it is offered in a genuine and loving fashion and we are always here to assist you. If you are having difficulties using your words ask your angels to step into your aura with you and guide you to communicate in a higher way.

Angel wisdom reminds you that communicating is a two way street so also listen with interest and respond openly, as this creates a bridge to others hearts and minds. Choose your words carefully and temper them with the love you have for this beautiful earth, your creator and yourself. Have faith and hope as being open brings you possibilities that you may not even see yet.

Affirmation: "I speak my truth from my heart. My words are filtered with love."

180

Look deeper

Find some quiet time to look within. Now is the perfect time to go within and contemplate where you have been and where it is you would like to go from here. Taking time and space for yourself gives you an opportunity to reflect on the way ahead, recoup from life's challenges, and prepare for the next phase in your life.

You are at the end of a cycle in your life. Call upon your angels to comfort you, and to guide you where you want to go to next. As you heal and move forward you are opening up to greater love, expansion and awareness. Stay the path which feels right in your heart, regardless what others may think, for this path will take you far, even if you can't see it yet. Ask your angels to help you feel strength, courage, and love anytime you need extra power.

Affirmation: "I take time for myself. I can clearly see the next best step for me."

181

Keep going

Keep charging ahead. You are almost there, don't turn back just yet. Sit by the side of the path for a bit if you feel you need to regain your footing, however the angels wish to remind you that now is the perfect moment to act upon your inspirations and charge ahead.

Expect miraculous solutions and situations to appear and more of them will begin to happen in your life. Everyone and everything is truly on your side. Know that you are worthy and deserving of all the beauty you desire, as is every other person doing the journey with you.

If you feel your confidence waiver, call us to your side and we will surround you with the love and strength to charge ahead.

Affirmation: "I trust in the Universe. I know the world is safe and working with me."

182

Fully supported

We hear your prayers for assistance and support. Ask your angels to help you heal any thoughts and emotions that are standing in your way. This assists in removing any blocks that stand between you and all that you desire to create. Open your heart to receiving. As you honour and follow the guidance of your heart, the more prosperity and abundance come your way.

Look at your belief systems about where you feel that you are blocked. Can you see where this was created? We are always with you to help and assist; this is why you came to do this journey with guardian angels by your side, so you would know that you are never alone and always supported. Just ask and we will go to work on your behalf, always, even if you don't feel it, trust that we are there. The more you release control and learn to trust, the more ideas, thoughts, feelings and knowingness will flow to you and through you.

Affirmation: "I am supported, I trust in the abundance of the Universe. I am deserving of all that I desire."

183

Power of joy

Joy is a high vibrating energy. When you fill your heart with laughter and joy, you fill each cell within your physical structure with highly charged particles of Divine Light which can be used in your manifestation process, healing, and transformation. This is a force that can help you transform any area of your life.

Angel wisdom reminds you to enjoy a good laugh. Work on projects that fill you with immense joy, and use this natural state of being to enhance all aspects of your life. When you are filled with these high vibrating particles you know that anything is possible.

Affirmation:"I am filled with joy and love, always."

184

The gift of change

Change brings great blessings and hope. Although lives sometimes feel turned upside-down, the changes that are occurring are divinely inspired by your asking. Changes help to release the energy that no longer serves your growth. Remember the Universe wants you to have your heart's desires. It is simply waiting for you to know and trust that you are worthy, and you are.

Do your part in deciding what you truly want. Then send out positive thoughts for the changes you seek and for the fulfillment of your wishes. Ask your angels for help and they will fan the sparks of potential and bring them into your life.

Angel wisdom reminds you that change brings in fresh opportunities to learn, grow, prosper, and create new relationships. The key is to keep breathing and enjoy the ride. Stay centered in the eye of the hurricane as the changes occur around and within you.

Affirmation: "I embrace the new in my life and choose peace as my guide."

185

Where are your thoughts

It is important to think about only what you truly desire, not what you fear. When you find that you are creating unwanted things in your life and you want to shout 'no', shout only briefly and then turn your focus to that which you desire to create. Any attention to anything is sending energy to that thought and will bring it to you.

Everything vibrates and is communicating, reacting and responding with everything around it. Once you begin to offer your energy on purpose, you then have absolute control of your experiences.

Angel wisdom reminds you that you cannot control others; you can control you and create in your own reality. Trying to limit others deifies the Laws of the Universe, it cannot be done. As you find harmony with your own desires, you are controlling and creating your own reality. You are never inhibiting or preventing anyone else from living the life they want to create for they too can only create in their reality.

Affirmation:"I am focusing on that which I desire; therefore I am attracting more of it into my life."

186

Day dream

Daydream regularly. Relax and open your mind. Connect to your still, quiet center and listen to the wisdom of your soul without directing your thoughts, as this more easily lets you hear and receive our messages. Notice your feelings, visions, and ideas. As you gain clarity you will more easily make decisions and act with truth and integrity from your own wise, infinite self.

After your visualization exercise, journal about the information that you received, as you do this your angels drop in all the information that you need to help you on your way. All that you receive in this short time is recorded in your mind. Just take the time to write it down and look at later.

Remember, happy outcomes follow positive expectations. Have patience and trust, and don't try to force things to happen. Relax, and be in a state of joy as you receive.

Affirmation: "I see happy outcomes for all that I desire."

187

Be strong

Be courageous. Hold your focus steadfastly. Everything can be yours; you can always be victorious, regardless of outside appearances. Ask your angels to step into your aura and support you during trying times, as these provide the best incidents for you to grow in leaps and bounds. This is why you agree to put them on your path. You always have a choice. If you have difficulty seeing the choices that are before you, ask us to assist your understanding.

Your angel guidance is to go into nature, preferable near water as water is a magnifier of energy, and also a cleanser, sweeping away debris and lower vibrating energy that can be picked up along the way. Close your eyes and connect to that still, quiet center within and hear the answers to your prayers. Allow your angels and the waters to cleanse you, ground you and return you to your center of balance and harmony.

Affirmation: "I am cleansed by the water beneath me. I can more easily connect and feel my guides and angels every day."

188

Patience

Your dreams are coming to fruition. Stay optimistic and remain positive. Follow your guidance and trust that your prayers are being answered. Detach from how they occur, be open to all the possibilities and know that if there seems to be a waiting period that we are lining up all the opportunities for you to experience. Like the director of a play, we set up situations based on your choosing and it is up to you to decide what direction you would like to go. Keep your mind and your heart open to the options that are available to your now.

Take an attitude of acceptance, relax and take stock while you are waiting. Know that we are indeed working diligently on your behalf. Don't give up. If you feel your confidence wavering, ask your angels to buoy your faith. For we are always with you, relax and feel safe, guided and comforted.

Affirmation: "I ask for what I desire. I am open to receiving in whatever form it appears for my highest good and the highest good of all."

189

Fresh air

A new outlook can be possible. Being in the beauty and splendour of Mother Nature can help to revive your spirit. Your cells are re-oxygenated by the grass, trees, plants, and flowers offering you healing and rejuvenation. Spend some time in the peace and tranquility that your beautiful earth offers you every day. When you take a moment to just breathe and be one with nature, your vibration is raised and you can more easily feel our presences and promptings.

When you emerge from your nature retreat pay attention to the signs and synchronicities and know that we place along your path as these are answers to your prayers. Trust that opportunities are available to you and start to expect and look for them and enjoy the divine timing of all things.

Affirmation: "Connecting with fresh air rejuvenates my cells and my outlook on life."

190

Creating loving unions

Focus on new beginnings within your relationships. Everyone has something to offer each situation, and as you learn to work together in harmony with each other, you can create in ways you have only previously dreamed about. Angel wisdom reminds you that together you are stronger. Each one carries a different piece of the puzzle, and as you fit these pieces together, you can create a picture of peace and harmony in these relationships and this changes all your other relationships too.

Take good care of yourself and each other and add a spiritual aspect to your work, play, and all your relationships. This helps bring that harmony and balance into the equation and adds to a desired outcome. Together you are stronger. Pay attention to your dreams, they are brilliant with symbols, and offer you a look at things without the mental energy of the ego.

The angels wish to remind you that life offers many shades of every colour, and these each have something wonderful to offer, so tap into the magic that each one brings with them.

Trust that you are creating in magical ways, trust your intuition to guide you in sensing what feels right and good, trust your judgment and then you are moving towards your dreams.

Affirmation: "My relationships are filled with love and with a spiritual foundation."

191

Adventure

Treat each day like a new adventure. Expect the unexpected and make the most of all the opportunities that are presented to you. Do things differently and approach life with a sense of wonder and awe.

If the path ahead seems dark or unsteady, ask your angels to light the way. Then watch for the signs that tell you which way to go next.

Explore the new with enthusiasm and courage and know that we are by your side to support you always. The angels are inspiring you to move forward with anticipation, expectancy and hope. These magnetic qualities attract the same, whether you desire to attract money, career opportunities or to add zest to your relationships.

Go outside and play today as this helps to create joy, and joy creates miracles and manifestations.

Affirmation: "I expect miraculous things to happen in my life, and they do."

192

Guardian Angels

You are never alone and we are always, always by your side. Each of you comes to this earth journey with an entourage of angelic helpers. The guardian angels are a group of angels who agree to assist and support the beautiful being of light that you are for your entire incarnation. They never leave you and are always by your side.

We are here to support you while you spiritually grow and

experience. We are here to help you in any way that supports your journey.

Spend some time getting to know your guardian angels and how we can help make your journey a more joyful, spirit filled experience. Quiet your mind and join with us, for we are closer to your vibration than other realms as we are always with you. Feel our love anytime you need support, or to just feel joy.

Our primary assignment is to be your support, please work more intimately with us and watch the miracles begin to occur.

Working with your Guardian Angels: We interact with many angels throughout our lifetime, and often we are not even aware of their assistance or energies as they are here solely to assist humanity in unconditional love of the Creator. Many angels come and go that work with us, the guardian angels that each one of us comes here with, stay with us for our entire life time. They are always with you. They do not judge, they only love us. You can talk with your guardian angels anytime.

Do a meditation and ask your angels what their names are and how you can work together with them. They absolutely love when we consciously interact with them.

Affirmation: "I can feel my support and connection with my guardian angels."

193

Renewed purpose

Trust and follow your renewed passion for life. The angels remind you that every situation or person is placed on your path for a purpose. It can be to bring you strength, opportunities, to release old patterns, or perhaps just to bring you joy. If your life is feeling like it is full of chaos and problems, look around and see the blessings within the circumstances, for these times are actually answers to your prayers. As you look more deeply into these patterns, they begin to dissolve and open up the new opportunities you have been asking for. Take care of the old to bring in the new.

There is help available to you in all realms. There are those in time and space with you who are there to support, love and guide you, just as our realm is here to do the same. Your angel guidance is to take some time to review where you've been and where you would like to go from here. Find the purpose in your current situations and then you are ready to move forward in the direction of your dreams.

Affirmation: "I am strong and determined and love the richness of my life."

194

Gratitude

Count your blessings. When you say thank you to the Universe, more is bestowed upon you. If you desire more love, offer more compassion for others. If you require more money, give graciously, and without expectation. Opening your heart is truly the first step. Honour yourself, for as you do this, it opens your heart to greater treasures.

Simplify your life in all ways possible. Give away things that you do not like, wear or want. Trust that the limitless supply of the Universe will provide what you need, when you need it. Be open to the many gifts in your life. Live in the present moment and trust that all is available to you. See the beauty that surrounds you. And know that we are always with you, holding your hand.

Affirmation: "I am grateful for everything in my life."

195

Spiritual growth

Opportunities for great change are available now. As you raise your vibrations, new psychic and spiritual experiences change the way you view yourself, life, the Universe and everything. Allow these gifts to open and expand. Use the power of study, prayer [the *asking*], and meditation [*the listening*] to expand your senses. Practice introducing new ways of being that bring you more peace and harmony. And, most importantly, have some fun along the way.

Use discernment. Remain positive and follow your guidance. Trust the still, quiet, and wise voice within you, for you are connected to every angel, guide, and the Creator always. Work with your higher, or authentic self always, for as you learn to trust yourself, your journey and how you view it will change.

Affirmation: "I trust my intuition. I choose for my greatest good."

196

Living your truth

You are guided to be true to yourself in all that you do. The angels say "Let go of anything unauthentic and all activities that do not mirror your highest intentions and desires for yourself." If there is something that is not working in your life at this time, be willing to release it and start again. You have the ability and power to turn all of your desires into reality.

When you release unhealthy situations, the energy begins to move, making way for Divine light to enter. You will find that 'the job, relationships, health issue, or other circumstances' heal in ways that you could never have imagined. The key is to trust that you are supported and release any thoughts of doubt or less than.

Hold feelings of joy in your heart. Joy is that magical sense that all things are possible, and they are. Appreciate the gifts within each moment.

Expect a miracle when you decide to be true to who you are.

Affirmation: "I live my life as my authentic self. I know that living my truth is the only way to be and experience the world."

197

Weighing your options

Make a list for the choices before you. Look deeper into your choices, that way, when you choose, you do so with clarity and commitment. We know that the Lightworkers greatest desire is to assist and create a 'better' world. This often leads to taking on more than your share. It is time to release that and take a good look at what it is you would truly like to focus and begin from there.

Ask your angels to be by your side, supporting you, and that you are aware of our presences and then be open to the thoughts, ideas, and words that come forth from your inner being. Ask us to step into your aura and help you see things from a different perspective, with the eyes of love.

Affirmation: "I carefully choose from all choices I have. I am connected to Divine guidance which always provides me with great options to choose from."

198

Play

It is time to set aside work for a while. Don't worry; we will oversee your responsibilities to their completion.

Angel wisdom shares that playfulness, gaiety, and laughter will lift your energy so that you'll come back with a renewed perspective and heightened energy for the tasks at hand.

Is your soul crying out for some fun? Feelings of fatigue, irritability, or depression are additional signs that you're overdue for some playtime. You don't need to wait until you have a free moment, because you can inject fun into your day today. Simple pleasures, moments of silliness, laughter with a friend, or watching a funny movie are good examples of ways to have fun that don't require a lot of time or money. Fun and play are necessary parts of life for children and adults. These types of activities help you live healthier lives, and allow you to attain our desires more quickly. Fun is part of living a balanced life.

Stop what you are doing and go have some fun right now. Release any guilt about having fun to the angels. You deserve happiness, pleasure and enjoyment. Make sure that you recreational activities are purely fun and non-competitive and if you can, play outside, breath fresh air, and feel the sun on your face (even if it is cloudy).

Affirmation: "I love to laugh and be in a state of joy and bliss and I can always choose to live my life this way."

199

Renewed purpose

Trust and follow your renewed passion for life. The angels remind you that every situation or person is placed on your path for a purpose. It can be to bring you strength, opportunities, to release old patterns, or perhaps just to bring you joy. If your life is feeling like it is full of chaos and problems, look around and see the blessings within the circumstances, as these times are actually answers to your prayers. As you look more deeply into these patterns, they begin to dissolve and open up the new opportunities you have been asking for. Take care of the old to bring in the new.

There is help available to you in all realms. There are those in time and space with you who are there to support, love and guide you, just as our realm is here to do the same. Your angel guidance is to take some time to review where you've been and where you would like to go from here. Find the purpose in your current situations and then you are ready to move forward in the direction of your dreams.

Affirmation: "I am strong and determined and love the richness of my life."

200

You are powerful

You are more powerful than you realize. Your inner power wants to surface. Your connection with the divine has become more powerful. During this time you are often filled with many different feelings, confusion, excitement, fear, and wonder. You want to be totally immersed in your spiritual life and studies, wishing you could read, study, learn, meditate, and do healings on a full time basis.

For some of you this is possible. Be sure to keep your focus and your thoughts on what you are creating. Trust that you are supported, loved, and guided each moment. Don't worry about how your future will blend with your spiritual growth.

Angel wisdom reminds you that if your focus is on, "What impact will my new spiritual pursuits have on my job, marriage, or friendships?" These worries create a fear that may erode the enjoyment your spiritual studies bring you. Surrender those feelings, as what you resist in life persists. Ask you angels to help you dissolve all the resistances of your ego (the inner conflict and struggle) so that we can help flood your life with higher truth and joy.

Begin taking small steps towards your goals of spiritual growth and understanding. Begin to focus on the service you can offer humankind at this stage in your evolution. Find ways that allow you to practice your growth and share your knowledge and allows you to be in your truth now, as well as to continue on your current path of growth and empowerment. As you begin to swim in the stream of your desires, on joyful service, you begin to feel that this stream continues to support your growth, and you begin to enjoy the shifts you see around you.

Use your power, talents, passions and interests to make the world a better place, put your focus on giving and receiving, then through the Law of Attraction, you'll receive all of the support you'll need.

Affirmation: "I am powerful. Being empowered is my natural state of being."

201

Surrender and release

We shower you with love and blessings. Open your arms and release the challenges you have held on to too tightly. Open your hands, arms, and heart to our love and assistance.

Angel wisdom reminds you that you are not alone and you don't need to try to fix everything by yourself. The angels are here and would love to help you and answer your prayers, first just surrender and release any situation that is holding you back. Surrender simply means that you are tired of the struggle. It means emotionally letting go, with trust that the Divine wisdom of Spirit can do the job. Surrender doesn't mean that you are giving up or that you want to be controlled. It means that through surrender, you'll release the burden and be open to ideas and thoughts of how to heal it. If you need help with surrender, ask your angels to assist you.

Release tension and any need to control, and things will open up and be better. Simply own your power and you won't have to fight it.

Affirmation: "I am powerful and creating that which I desire."

202

Set your sights higher

What is it you truly desire?

Expect the most for yourself, don't settle. Shoot for the stars, and trust that your desires will be fulfilled. This is an opportunity of tremendous growth and change. What is paramount is that you desire it fully and completely and then get out of the way and do your work. We shall do ours. Of course you need to invoke us. Which means, invite us into your experience. And for you to remember that you can have it all.

This is a great time to sign up for a new course that assists in your growth and evolution. It is a time to let go of the past and expect different results that you have previously expected and watch how your world begins to shape into something entirely new and exciting. The past weights you down, let it go now. Imagine your wildest dreams coming true and then work at feeling that every day.

Affirmation: "I am ready to move forward and expand my light."

203

Wait

Bide your time until you feel confident in your journey. You don't necessarily need to feel full confidence, however believe in the possibility of your dreams. In fact we prefer it if there is a little apprehension as it shows you are evolving beyond your comfort zone. And you should feel a bit of that, or perhaps the task at hand is not helping you grow. All circumstances you find yourself in are designed to help you grow. Be it a relationship, a career, a hobby, or a trait in yourself, they are here to help you grow. It can be to grow in love, in joy, in being in the movement and appreciating all the gifts you already have.

There no accidents along the way. Everything and everyone is orchestrated, like a movie, to assist you in your soul's growth.

Angel guidance suggests that you don't need to rush forward; all things can wait for you, take some quiet time and connect with your guidance, and then if you need to, gather more information. Then when you feel confident or are able to fully trust and take the next step. There is no race, no need to hurry. Stop along the way and relax, sing by a fire, and enjoy all the gifts you have and have been given on your journey.

There are no wrong turns.

Affirmation: "I have all the time I need to accomplish all I want to do."

204

Peace

Be at peace, regardless where you are. There is no need to worry, as everything will work out beautifully, even if you perhaps can't see that yet. There are no accidents in your linear world, trust and infuse love into all that you do. Regardless as to where you are or what is happening in your life, take a moment and sit back and infuse love to all of those involved. Envision all the right people be in the right place to have this taken care of quickly and as painlessly as possible for everyone involved, and then release it, do what you need to do and move on. Expect miraculous solutions to appear, and they indeed will.

And, accept where you are with unconditional love for yourself or others. The angels ask you to remember to accept everyone exactly as they are, without judging, blaming or wanting to change them. Accept, which is to unconditionally love them. Let your true self emerge and be love.

Affirmation: "I love and accept all things, regardless as how they appear."

205

Focus on service

Feed your soul by being of service. You are needed to shine your light. If you feel you are unable to be your true self in all parts of your life, find something to do that feeds your soul. Volunteer at the food bank, animal shelter, hospital, hospice, church, theatre, school, or wherever your heart feels expressed. Light is needed in so many areas that it is too big to write them all out. Not everyone is able to immediately make a living being in their purpose. What is most important is to accept where you are, and immerse yourself as much as possible in pursuits that bring you absolute joy.

Make time in your life for anything that brings joy to your soul. That is the first step towards creating a blissful life. Release any thoughts that are old and outdated. This sometimes is a challenge, especially if you have carried this thought since childhood or over many lifetimes. Ask your angels to help you remove these thoughts from your cellular DNA, in all dimensions of time and space, and we will begin to help you and or lead you to a healer who can. Be open to receive, open your heart and feed your soul.

Affirmation: "Being in service to humanity makes my soul sing."

206

Inner peace

Inner peace is your natural state.

It brings you a new tranquility and a smoother road ahead. Spend time alone where you can relax your mind, body and spirit. From this place of peace, allow the energy to flow into all aspects of your being and then let it flow into every corner of your life. Fill every nook and cranny with love and our light. And, when you return to the real world once again you will feel that state of being that you have when you are not in physicality that so many of you long to feel. It is yours and is available to you always.

Foster your skills, talents and passions for the good of yourself and all. Eliminate power struggles, conflicts, and competition, as these are old energy thoughts that there is not enough for everyone. The purpose of live is to joyfully serve and to swim in a stream of great joy and bliss. Find those activities that best mirror what you want to create in the world.

Angel wisdom reminds you that through breath and intention, you can stay centered. This foundation of inner peace has a powerful healing affect and will soon be reflected in your outer world.

Affirmation: "I am at peace. I am filled with a tranquility and peace of mind which is my divine birthright."

207

Notice the light

Ask for us to light your way. The angels will always lead you toward the answer to your prayers. Listen and follow the steps that we communicate through your thoughts, intuition and dreams. We cannot assist you until we are asked and we don't do the journey for you, we light the path that is of your asking.

Quiet your mind and body, tap into the unlimited force of nature and connect with your guides and angels. Ask us what is the next best step for you take that brings you closer to your ultimate destination. We will light the way, often ever so subtly, that it brings you closer to your desire. Clarity on what you choose to experience is paramount in providing us with the best information to assist you. We see only love and your evolution in all things. We do not choose for you, for that is purpose of free will. Free will is the immutable law of the Earth experience.

Trust that we are there and lighting your path and you will actually see light before you, guiding you. Trust that we are with you and feel our love and compassion and support for you on your journey. All are on your side, even if you can't see or feel that yet.

Affirmation: "My path in life is bright and the lighted path is obvious before me."

208

Take action

Take action gently, and with love. Trust your instincts and lovingly assert yourself to heal any situations that are in need of healing. Strength and truthfulness are paramount in ensuring the best possible outcome for all. Ask your angels to stand with you as you speak your truth. We can give you strength, and guide your words so that feelings won't be hurt. And if they are, we wish to remind you that when you speak your truth with love and compassion, you have done your part. It is up to the recipients to realize your intentions when they are ready to do so. You cannot change another, only yourself and how you view the situation.

Have faith, remain positive and follow your inner guidance. There are no wrong turns, just sometime longer paths to get where you want to go. Trust that you are exactly where you want to be right now and from that point, take the next step. Trust yourself; do not put blind faith in another, only in yourself. And know that you are never alone and we are always by your side. Call to us and we are there. It is that simple.

Affirmation: "I am strong, compassionate, and speak my truth from my heart."

209

A new day

Tomorrow is a new day. New opportunities are available to you with each new sunrise. The worst is now behind you, and positive new experiences are on the horizon. Don't give up just as you are about to cross a huge hurdle in your life. We know it is not always easy to do a human journey and that many times it seems that there is no choice other than to give up. Your angels surround you with love and hold you so tight during those dark hours, and in the morning a fresh new perspective is always available to you. Take time to relax, be still, and feel much needed care from us. Remember the Universe wants you to have everything that you desire and that there is something more coming up before you.

Keep your thoughts positive, use affirmations and carry them with you when you feel your spirit wane. Take time to see the beauty that surrounds you, in the trees, in the hearts of children, in the hearts of those you hold dear. Keep hope in your heart dear ones, and feel the love and honour that we bestow upon you.

Affirmation: "I am eternally optimistic. I know that wonderful things are happening for me now."

210

Laughter

Laughter is the best medicine. Laughter is a wonderful healer. Let it help you heal. Sometimes a situation cannot heal until you release the challenge completely so that healing light can enter. Do not focus on what went wrong, focus on what went right and what the gift is within the situation and know that it is time to let it go. Do something today that makes you laugh, and as you forget any troubles or confusion and release that energy; your angels can drop in suggestions that let you see things from a different light.

Know that Archangel Michael is always available to offer guidance and protection, invoke him often. Do not worry that you are asking too much. The angels are not ground to time and space and can be with everyone who calls upon them. Use the power of laughter and friendship in your healing. Laughter is the sunshine that dissolves the darkness, so make merry, and have some fun. And, Laugh often and Laugh loudly.

Affirmation: "I love to laugh and enjoy my life."

211

Let your spirit be free

Be true to your thoughts and feelings. See the beauty that surrounds you and know that it is time to fulfill that which is in your heart and is your passion. There is a longing within each soul who is not expressing themselves in their highest light. There is an underlying current of dissatisfaction, no matter how successful that person is, within them if they are not honouring what they came here to accomplish. Everything that you do in your life is by choice and the angels wish to remind you that it is okay to choose again.

Work very closely with your angels during times of transition. Surrender any guilt or other negative emotions you might be carrying around to us and let us assist you in your transformation. Know that endings are beginnings and each phase of your life is a new cycle. Use the energy of your longing to create and focus on freeing your soul. Be kind to yourself and let your spirit be free.

Affirmation: "My spirit if free; I see beauty all around me."

212

Meditation

Meditation is a most important tool. Practice it often. Quiet your mind and hear the voices of your angels and guides. Meditation allows your angels to interact with you, answer your questions, as well as bring you peace, tranquility and healing.

Spend at least 5 minutes each morning with your eyes closed, focus on your breath for a few minutes, and then ask us a question, or something you would like clarity on and just relax and listen. Don't try too hard or be too hard on yourself at first, just continue to breathe in and out deeply, slowly and relax.

Release thoughts that you don't need and enjoy these experiences. We eagerly await our connection and communication together.

Affirmation: "I easily connect with guides and angels and interpret the messages I receive."

213

What do you desire

You now have the opportunity to write the script. What do you desire?

Now is the time to decide what you really want to manifest in your life, using your determination to manifest results in the physical world. You need to take control, grab those reins and move forward, and be sure you are heading in the direction in which you wish to go. Protect yourself against negativity at this time as it is often easy to become distracted and/or discouraged by other peoples thoughts and desires for you. Instead, focus on your dreams and get inspired, then move determinedly toward that which you desire to create. Be a resolute and gentle warrior.

Angel wisdom reminds you that it is inspiring when you start to take real control of your life. Meditate, keep calm, and take what action you feel guided to take. Wear blinders to naysayers and sceptics. It is your life, work on changing it for yourself and no one else. It really doesn't matter what others think or feel about what course you take, it matters how you think and feel. If you feel you cannot change things at this moment, work on changing how you feel about it. You always have a choice, and it is perfectly acceptable to choose again. See the gifts in what you have learned and experienced and offer gratitude for all that you have been through, for it is those things that make you who and what you are.

You are dearly loved for whatever road you take, the choice is always yours, what do you truly desire to manifest in your life!

Affirmation: "I am in control of my destiny; I am focused on creating that which I desire."

214

Be true to yourself

It is time to be your authentic self. Make your real feelings and beliefs your truth. Share with others who you truly are. Let people see your true nature. Let people feel your wisdom; let them feel your love. Follow what lies in your heart. Live your truth, as you are a most beautiful part of the creator, and all that is.

Your relationships will change when you 'come out of the closet'. Those that aren't evolving will naturally drop away, and other relationships will deepen as you will know that you are loved for who you truly are. Love yourself. Trust and follow your intuition. You can be divinely guided, for you can always tap into the wellspring of infinite knowledge. Trust the knowingness, the visions, or the inner voice that is trying to share with you to enhance your journey. Know that you are spiritual supported in this process by the guides and the angels.

Use positive affirmations each day to assist you in all that you wish to create and manifest. This is a powerful tool should you choose to use it. Before or immediately after arising, spend a few minutes thinking about your desires. Allow yourself to imagine that they've already manifested. Set your intention for what you would like to create in your day today (each day). And, as you go about your day, let go of any judgments about yourself or others. Speak your truth with **LOVE**. Allow others to get to know the real you.

Affirmation: "I speak my truth from my heart. I follow my inner guidance at all times."

215

Signs

We are sending you signs. Coincidences and synchronicities are carefully orchestrated by your guides and angels, as you have asked, so pay careful attention to the messages that are all around you.

There is no such thing as chance, in your amazing Universe. We carefully plan each phase of your journey with your guides and angels and your higher self, and they cleverly deliver you the signs and synchronicity on your path. There might be a bird or a butterfly that flies near you to let you know that they are working with you, working for you. You may hear a song several times that means something to you or makes you think of someone, or perhaps even helps you release and grow. Signs are plentiful and all around you.

Pay attention to the messages and signs that come your way, as these are guideposts to assist you on your path. If you ask the angels for a sign, or have a question or a decision to make, be open to receiving it, don't specify what sign you would like to receive, leave that up to your angels.

Start to expect and look for the signs. Be aware that there is a divine reason behind them and consider what the message or lesson is. Rejoice when you notice them, offer gratitude and know that you deserve to receive good in all ways.

Affirmation:"All things happen in divine order. I easily notice the signs that are all around me."

216

Letting go

Release any worries or powerless thoughts, as these could be holding you back. If you are attached to people, things, or circumstances that are not of a high vibration, it is time to release them. If you are holding expectations of others to make things better, it is time to release this also, as it holds you to a lower frequency that can keep you stuck where you are.

Your angel guidance is to ask your angels to help you cut the cords that tie you to people, things and emotions. When these are released, you can reclaim your power. Trust your intuition; listen to your higher self. You will do the right thing for all concerned, even if this is indeed the hardest choice you have to make.

Affirmation:"I release everyone and everything. My spirit is free."

217

Trust

Trust in yourself. Trust that you do indeed deserve it all. This is one of the most difficult tasks many face. Sometimes when humans have trusted, they have felt let down, first by others and then themselves. The angels wish to remind you to begin again fresh and new. If you are holding on to past experiences and old results, you will get more of the same. That is the Universal Law of Attraction. It is therefore important for you to focus on what is happening now and what is currently before you, and not keep looking in the past.

Put your faith in yourself. Listen to your intuition; listen to the emotions that come from your heart. Ask us to help you release any fears that might be blocking you from enjoying unconditional trust in yourself.

Let your angels flood you with their love and allow it to flow into your heart and your mind. Clear old thought patterns and ask us to help you to release them. Allow yourself to spontaneously feel the love, and trust that you are powerful and deserving.

Affirmation: "I trust in my ability of discernment. I listen and trust my intuition more and more each day."

218

Stay optimistic

Ground yourself with Mother Earth. When all around you seems to be falling apart, take a breath, and connect with your beautiful Terra.

In these changing times that you are amidst, remember to stay optimistic and ground yourself regularly. Use the power of affirmations to keep your focus, and your conscious connection with Mother Earth will help you to keep that focus.

Sometimes humans get detached from the very earth they live on when they are doing higher work, and in these days of higher energy, many want to be detached. However the angels want to remind you that you are here doing a physical journey, and as you learn to work with these higher energy times, you will find that you are more able to create that which you desire. Grounding yourself while you work with this energy assists in creating your dreams in the 3D world.

So, talk positively, focus on the good in life and feel happier and healthier in the process.

Affirmation: "I cherish and nurture Mother Earth, and she cherishes and nurtures me."

219

Reward yourself

Take the time to reward yourself. Do something for yourself in a meaningful way. Keep your faith strong in creating that which you desire. In order for you to keep your reserves high, take excellent care of yourself. You are an important gift and have unique attributes that only you can offer at this time and we pledge to you to share your gifts with others. Take time out regularly to treat yourself as special as you would a dear friend. Ask a dear friend to join you and create joy together. You are always stronger in greater numbers.

Have faith and hope that your dreams are manifesting, even if you can't see it yet. There is always a blessing in each situation. See that blessings and release it. To manifest more rapidly, think of that which you desire while playing music, chanting or humming. This increases the resonance of the dream and the dreamer. Dream Big!

Affirmation: "The Universal supply is unlimited and I am entitled to all the beauty, bounty and abundance that are available to everyone."

220

Dreams of change

The changes you have been dreaming of are manifesting in your reality. As you focus on that which you want to change, you are experiencing true growth. You may have felt you have had a bumpy ride in the beginning of your shift and as this shift continues, with your resolute focus, you will know that it truly is a ride you were meant to take and enjoy the new way of being that has resulted from these changes.

You may have been questioning aspects of your life over the last little while, at the very least you've been dreaming of wider pastures, treasure chests filled with booty, or becoming a stronger force, as you take your power. Whatever your have been longing to create in your life, NOW is the time to step up the energy as you are moving closer to creating that which you have been dreaming of creating for yourself. Keep your focus and keep moving. This will attract the right people, business, and love that you have been working for.

The angels wish to remind you that destiny is the trip you take to get there, not the destination.

Affirmation: "I am free to choose and focus my attention on that which I desire."

221

Patience

Be patient with yourself. You are a beautiful being of Creator energy that is learning to be finite. This is no small task and we honour you who have stepped up into your contracts, often with such great zeal.

We are honoured to be your guidance. Take time out each day to feel our love for you, it will do wonders in buoying your energy and strength. Angel wisdom reminds you that love is the underlying energy of every situation on your earth plane. Therefore we ask that you see only love and infuse only love into all that you do. As you bring more love into all that you do, you will receive rewards in undreamed of way.

Take each step with thoroughness of thought, and conviction. As you focus on working towards that which lies in your heart, you cannot help but create in your life. Are you ready? We are always with you, by your side. Please invoke us and let us all be of service at this wonderful time on your planet.

Affirmation: "Everything unfolds exactly as it should; I see the love that is all around me and in all that I do."

222

Freedom

Your spirit longs to be free. It is felt deeply, as you have the stirring memories of freedom within you. As you connect with and trust your connection with us and the Divine, you feel your connection with your higher or authentic self. As you connect more frequently and trust that part of you that is not bound by time and space, you once again feel the freedom of soul. You will realize that you are indeed infinite and bound by only your thoughts of less than.

Each of you has an important purpose at this time, even if you are not sure what it is. Your purpose is always changing, just as you are and so therefore we ask you to think of what you can do now to bring about the earth plane changes that are necessary at this time. As you release the need to be in service with the joy of being in service, this is when you tap into the energy of passion. Live your passion in whatever way you can at this time. Connect with your higher self and feel the merge that is taking place with the finite and the infinite and watch your world change.

Affirmation: "I release any limits to my freedom. I am in charge of my life."

223

Love

Strive to feel love. Wherever you are, whatever you are doing, feel love. Feel love for your fellow travelers, regardless as to where they may be. Feel love for yourself and the choices you have made. Feel love for all as you go about your daily tasks, even if you don't particularly like whom they currently are or what they are doing. Fill your heart with compassion, and love them anyway.

There is plenty of opportunity to share love on your beautiful planet, and plenty of opportunity to grow. Embrace all that is around you. It is through love that you will change your world. Change the world with your smile. Share your life, share your love.

Affirmation: "I am surrounded by loving people, and places. I am love, and it is felt by others in my smile and seen in my eyes."

224

Finding balance

Take a deep breath and find your center. Once you are there, ground your energy first with the Earth, and then with the stars, and then blend your heart with ours. From this still point of reference all things are possible. There is no doubt or fear here, for it cannot exist in the presence of love.

It is important to connect with Earth as a regular part of your spiritual practice. It will help you keep your center and be in balance. Nature offers so many gifts that will open up to those who are brave enough to dare. Realize that your experiences on your Earth journey are about finding the joy of being in each moment, regardless. We applaud you for having the courage to do so without the memories to your magnificence and you are each awakening to that daily.

Affirmation: "I connect my heart with that of the earth, and that of the stars, and that of the Divine Creator, and find my balance in this with me as the center of the trinity."

225

Worry not

Let your focus be on your desires. If you are spending time worrying if you will have enough, if there is enough for everyone or will someone else get more, then your focus is on lack and you will therefore attract more of the same toward yourself. Your angel guidance is to keep you focus on your desires, on how you will feel having achieved that desire, and trusting that the signs will appear along the way and that you will indeed notice these signs.

Trust is a big part of the human journey. Trust that you can and will manifest your desires in undreamed of ways and that more will come your way than you could possibly imagine. Hold this thought as your truth often and watch as your life changes. You have fought the good fight; it is now time to revel in the rewards of your perseverance.

Release any worries or stress that you have about creating, as this will release a huge block in what you wish to manifest. Trust that new and better things are on the way.

Affirmation: "I release all limitations. I live in a limitless world."

226

Explore

It is time for your life to flow. Take the time to explore the different options that are available to you and see what each one might look like. Which one gives you the best feelings of love and joy? And then, from that place of least resistance you can clearly move forward. As humans, the lessons are often learned faster in a time of chaos or crisis; however it doesn't have to be that way.

Angel guidance reminds you that you always have time, it is

never wrong, and you are always surrounded by love. To feel the love that surrounds you, open your heart. To feel love for another, open your heart. To feel balanced and joyful, open your heart. You get the picture. All things can be solved from the point of unconditional love. Start small and expand as you move forward with spiritual confidence. Very soon you will have noticed the world around you has changed.

Affirmation: "I am free to choose. I see the path clearly ahead of me with each step I take. I am clearly hearing, feeling and knowing my connection to my inner wisdom so I can eagerly explore my life."

227

Power of love

You are reminded that your very essence is love and that love is a powerful energy. Open your heart center and share your love with everyone and everything. This does not mean that you do whatever they ask of you, it means that you unconditionally accept them, without judgment, without expectation. Each of you has the power of the Creator within you. All the power of Divine love, wisdom, and intelligence is available to everyone. Choose to be Love.

When you feel that love, you feel serene and at peace, you are powerful. You have the spiritual power to communicate with us and receive guidance. Tap in to the universal wisdom of the One Mind, empathize with others and remember that you are truly unlimited.

The more you open your heart, the more Love, Peace and Joy you feel and live.

Affirmation: "I am serene, powerful and confident, I am Love."

228

Release the past

It is time to let go of past hurts, regrets, and unfinished business. Some of this process might seem painful and difficult; however it is worth the journey to the other side.

There are actions and people from the past that you are being urged to gently let go of. Soon enough the purpose or this process, as difficult as it may seem at the time, will become clear and you will understand that in order to grow and evolve, this process and the energy it creates is destiny working its magic. The process of change will help to create the energy and strength for new projects, new loves, new friends and a new life.

Angel wisdom reminds you that as you release the past, you can build a better and stronger future, with or without certain people or situations in your life. This is a great time to seek out true friends, and you know there are a couple of people in this world that you trust beyond others. Now is that time to cultivate those contacts. This process makes way for the new, desired energy you long to create.

Affirmation: "I release the past; I seek out new experiences and infuse love into all that I do."

229

Make a wish

This can be a magical time. Trust that you can have all that you need to create all that you desire. No one will face lack because your dreams come true. There is enough for everyone in this infinite Universe. After you make your wish, look for the signs of which way to go next. Use your heart as your guide and feel your way along. Keep your thoughts positive and avoid the sceptics in your life.

You are protected from all types of harm. We ask that you relax and feel safe. Enjoy your journey for it truly is a beautiful world. Do not put your focus on things that appear to have gone wrong, for this adds that energy to the situation. When you keep your thoughts focused and positive, that is the energy you draw to you. Keep your heart full and trust that all is as it should be. As each of you learns to trust and love, that is when you will see your world changing into the era of peace, love and harmony for all.

Affirmation: "I know there is enough for everyone in this unlimited Universe."

230

Compassion

Soften your heart to everyone and everything, especially yourself. Work at forgiving yourself, and seeing your actions from a higher perspective. As you do this, you see the actions of others in a new light. As you develop compassion, others will naturally follow as they see you learn to live your life from the perspective of compassion. It is a powerful tool of spiritual growth. You don't need to change your stance or behaviour; it simply means that you can approach life with a loving heart.

See yourself and others through the eyes of your angels, with unconditional love and acceptance, regardless as to how it appears at first. The more love and compassion you begin to feel, the more the things around you seem to change. Yet it is truly you seeing the world from a higher perspective and allows any troubles, difficult relationships and lower energies to be transformed.

Affirmation: "I am cleansed with the Magenta flame and my heart is filled with compassion."

231

Release

Put down your burdens. Release that which you no longer need or want. Say no to things that you do not need to do. Let others do what their responsibility and let them be responsible

Sharon Taphorn

for themselves. You are not responsible for the actions of those around, only yourself and how you respond to them. Set healthy boundaries for yourself of what is acceptable and what is not. Decide what your responsibility is and what is theirs, and firmly set your course. You are helping to empower them by allowing them to do their own work. You are helping yourself by releasing the heavy burdens that you carry with you.

Take some time to get away from it all, even if it is just for an afternoon. Go somewhere that is pristine and quiet and just be in the moment of the beauty that surrounds you. Let Mother Nature cradle you in her arms and soothe your heart. This will allow inspiration and hope to return to your life. The wisdom you gain from this sojourn is exactly what the angels prescribe.

Make the commitment today to honour yourself and release the need to carry the world on your shoulders.

Affirmation: "I release the need to do everything by myself; each of us has a vital role to play in the game of life and honour everyone for all that they do. I honour myself."

232

Purposeful action

Move forward on purpose, not by default. Decide where you want to put your energy and then trust that it can all be created and, follow your heart, follow your passion. It is time to create the changes and results that you long for in your heart. When you clearly focus on your desires and take the steps you are guided to take, the path flows more smoothly. There is less juggling and wondering what will happen next. Instead you flow towards your desires.

This is a time of great change. Decisions that can alter the path of your life are before you now. Your light and your gifts are needed and serve as a beacon for those who are just awakening. You lead by example, and it is now time to step forward more fully into your passions.

Affirmation: "I direct the flow in my life. By following my passions, I create the life I desire."

233

Peace and serenity

Serenity, love, tranquility and peace are qualities worth cultivating. The angels in turn ask you to spread these beautiful qualities to others. Let this be a time of new beginnings and look to the past as a blessing in your evolution. Angel wisdom reminds you that you wouldn't be where you are now if it weren't for all that you have been through. So, celebrate who you are and who you are becoming, for you are indeed a beautiful light that does make a difference in the world.

Peace and serenity can be yours in every situation. There isn't a time when you don't have a choice about how you approach anything or any task, regardless of what is happening around you. Take a moment, close your eyes, take a deep breath and focus on your heart. Imagine that you are encircled in golden light of the sun and that this orb helps to keep your energy clear and bright. Feel the love of your angels and use this energy to beam to others around you.

Affirmation: "I am one with everyone in peace, love, and serenity."

234

Surround yourself with positive energy

Surrounding yourself with positive people and situations allows you to attract and create your intentions and future moments in their highest potentials.

Angel wisdom suggests that you use your skills and talents with intention. Eliminate power struggles, conflicts and competition, which comes from the mental body. This promotes harmony and joy around you and a magical sense that all things are possible. Appreciate the gifts within each moment and attract and create all that you desire.

Avoid negative people, situations, and influences as much as possible. Avoid negative discussions with yourself and others turn off programs with negative themes, and stay away from violent movies, avoid gossip magazines and programs. This will assist you in cleansing any hidden blocks that could slow you down from manifesting the results you desire.

Affirmation: "I am surrounding by loving thoughts about myself and others, I am light."

235

Beginnings

Life happens in cycles. There is a time of rebirth always happening. Do not be afraid to let go of that which is familiar, for the new cannot enter until the old has been released. Your angel guidance is to allow the new into your life when it arrives, and say a happy farewell to the old. You are protected always, so trust that new will bring you more that you can possibly imagine.

If those around you seem unhappy or threatened by the expansion of who you are, it is truly because they think they are protecting you in some way and it is an act of love. Soon, they will see you and things in a different light and your strength and courage helps to inspire others to take their power and step purposefully into their contracts. See the love in all things and keep your focus on your journey.

Ask and be open to receiving our support for we are always there when you call.

Affirmation: "I am open and receptive to new experiences, situations, people and activities."

236

Innocence

Recall your innocence. For everyone is a beautiful spark of Creator energy. Remember the beautiful innocence of a child and the wonder with which they view the world and then cultivate these qualities within you once again. Then, begin to explore the world once again from this beautiful perspective of spirit.

Imagine that each butterfly is the first one you have ever seen. Smell the flowers as if it is your first time enjoying their scent and beauty. Let the wave's crash against your feet and imagine that it too is the very first time. See the wonder and the beauty that surrounds you and then feel it with your heart. See it with your heart, feel it with all of your senses and be one with all that surrounds you.

Affirmation: "I see my world through the wonder of a child. I am surrounded by love and beauty always."

237

Acknowledge

Look after yourself. Acknowledge your desires and needs, then takes steps to meet them. Take a look at all the gifts you have to offer and acknowledge your talents and achievements. Also become aware of these qualities in those around you, for this brings more of that energy to you and also to them.

See and share who you truly are. You and every other living thing on the earth plane are made up of beautiful particles of Creator light. Let that beautiful light shine forth for others to see and be guided by. Bloom where you grow and watch the miracles that occur around you at every moment. Focus on what you can do right now to cultivate and support this energy and let your spirit soar.

Affirmation: "I acknowledge who I really am. My spirit is free."

238

Inner guidance

Tune into your guidance. Take time to pause, reflect and observe what follows when you trust your innate knowledge. It is your birthright to connect to, and follow that guidance. This is part of your evolution and all have access to all knowledge that exists in all realms. The challenge is in trusting what you receive and ensuring that you are tuning into the inner aspects of self and not into the mental energy of your mind.

Take a moment and quiet yourself and your thoughts, feel the love that flows up within you as you ask to connect with your authentic self and higher wisdom, and from this point of love, trust the stillness, trust that all is available to you. We are here by your side, loving and supporting you as well as offering you guidance. We are a part of you and stand ready and waiting for your beckoning call.

Trust that you are dearly loved, dearly supported and that your wise, loving center is open and encircling you with the wisdom of the Divine.

Affirmation: "Everything in my life is bringing me to a higher level of evolution."

239

You are safe

You are always protected against lower energies. Call upon Archangel Michael when you need help with courage or to assist in the release of fear and other lower thought forms. As you make changes in your life and as you encounter challenges, know that you are always safe and secure.

Have a heart to heart discussion with Archangel Michael often. Pour out all of your concerns to him. Don't worry about overburdening him, as Michael, like all other archangels, is able to be with everyone simultaneously who calls upon him. He has no limitations of time and space, so he can help everyone anytime they ask.

If you become worried or anxious, call in Michael to bring you peace. He can also help you clear the energy in your home, office, vehicle, or community, removing toxic energies like a chimney sweep. When Michael is near you'll likely notice a warm glow in your cheeks or perhaps see sparks of royal blue light. You can ask Michael to stay with you continuously if you feel the need, as he is able to be with everyone who calls upon him.

Call on Archangel Michael, and let his mighty sword cut any cords that bind you to others or lower energies. You will feel better regardless of what is happening around you.

Affirmation: "I am safe and protected always."

240

Listening

Quiet your mind, take some deep breaths, and listen to the quiet voices of love. Trust that you are hearing our messages. Let us reassure you that everything is taken care of, you are safe, and dearly loved. Everything is in Universal order and therefore filled with Divine love. Infuse only loving thoughts and emotions into every aspect of your life to ensure that the highest possible outcome flows effortlessly to and through you.

Stay in a quiet and receptive state. Focus on the next step on your path of manifestations, not the exact nature you think should happen, instead be open to the magnificent possibilities that are before you. Your quiet mind and body hears us more quickly and clearly. Let us surround you in the Creators love and listen to the promptings of the Divine.

Affirmation: "Each day I am hearing my guidance clearer and clearer. I am in the flow of my Divine connection."

241

Relationships

The most important relationship you have is with yourself. All other relationships flow from this energy. How do you feel about yourself? It is safe for you to explore and cultivate your many selves, your higher self and how you feel about them.

The relationships in your lives are vast and many. If there is an imbalance in your relationship with yourself, it is reflected in your relationships with others. Spend time getting to know and love yourself. What qualities do you love about yourself? What don't you love about yourself? Focus on your wonderful qualities and work on loving the ones you don't, as well as the ones you would like to have.

Angel wisdom reminds you that you are truly a beautiful and special person. You are worthy of healthy, balanced relationships, and to trust in yourself to make wise and honourable decisions. Most often blocks in attracting or healing relationships are rooted in an emotional experience from childhood or within a past or existing relationship. Ask your inner child what relationships mean to you in general and/or a specific relationship so that you can better understand and heal. Then, in your mind and your heart, surround yourself, the situations, and the person(s) with calming pink light and ask the angels to help you. Be open to the gifts within each situation and allow yourself to feel the love and peace once again.

Affirmation: "I am love, I am loveable, and I am loved."

242

Positive energy

Surround yourself with desired energy. Surround yourself with people who support you, make you smile and make you laugh whenever possible. This energy makes it easier to attract and create your intentions and future moments in their highest potential.

Angel wisdom suggests that you use your skills and talents with intention. This promotes harmony and joy around you and a magical sense that all things are possible. Appreciate the gifts within each moment and this will allows you to more easily attract and create all that you desire.

Avoid negative people, situations, and influences as much as possible. Avoid negative discussions with yourself and others, turn off programs with negative themes, and stay away from violent movies etc. This will assist you in cleansing any hidden blocks that could slow you down from manifesting the results you desire. Eliminate power struggles, conflicts and competition, which come from an ego desire to win.

Affirmation: "I am surrounding by loving thoughts about myself and others, I am light."

243

As you believe, so shall it be

You are more powerful than you may realize. Ask yourself "What is it I believe?" Angel wisdom reminds you that it is important to think about what you want, not what you don't want. Guard your thoughts as these are the very thoughts that are creating your current and future experiences. Our thoughts always have an effect, ALWAYS, and there are no neutral thoughts. You can learn to monitor and alter your thoughts.

Examine where your belief systems are in correlation to what you are receiving and desiring. This is the first step. The next step is to transform those belief systems to match the current you. Many belief systems are out of date and need to be updated to match the latest and always changing vibration of you.

Affirmation: "I am now able to focus my mind at will. I hold only loving thoughts, and my angels are gatekeepers in establishing a steady stream of thoughts with love and compassion."

244

Love for animals

Learn to connect with the Kingdom of the animals. Each animal has something to teach and share. Dogs in particular are about showing humans what unconditional love is. They do not judge you; they just love you, and can be a source of love and joy. Just as you can hear what your angels are saying, if you sit quietly, turn on your heart energy; you will receive images and feelings from your animals. If the animal has been mistreated, it might take a little longer for them to share with you. However if you let your heart energy flow all around you, they will eventual come to you. Sometimes it takes time. They respond to love.

Every animal of the earth has something to share and contribute. Share your gratitude with them. Let them know you are just as grateful to them for joining you on this journey, even if you do not understand why it is there. Accept that each one, including your creepy crawlers, has a purpose and a point to sharing the planet. And that you are all a part of grander plan than you can possibly imagine.

Just like the trees and the skies, they have a right to be here. Cherish them as you do one another.

Affirmation: "I love and appreciate all aspects of the earth experience."

245

A new dawn

Positive new experiences are on the horizon. New abundances and exciting opportunities are available to you right now! The worst is now behind you and it is time to move forward and choose to see the gift in your current circumstances and move beyond them now. What may have seemed like a dark time in your life has the opportunity to bring in the light, let it shine as bright as you can possibly make it and make room for creative ideas to enter.

Reward yourself by balancing your giving and receives. The angels wish to remind you that balancing your giving and receiving is essential for keeping your energy, mood and motivation at a consistently high level.

Affirmation: "Waves of prosperity and new experiences are coming my way now."

246

Enchantment

Life can be electrifying as its very essence is energy.

The angels ask you to recapture that magical sense that everything is possible and that a miraculous power surrounds you. Magic energy is available to everyone and not just a select few. It is just that some believe they are not worthy. Release any doubts or thoughts of less than and know you are deserving of all that you desire.

Your angel guidance is to take some contemplation time meditating upon what you truly desire. When you are truly clear on what you want, your angels can see the energy of your desires and doors begin to open as you attract this energy to you.

Affirmation: "I picture my desired outcomes and I am now bringing my dreams into physical manifestation."

And trust that it is so dear ones!

247

Divine order

You have the power and support to make desired changes in your life right now.

Your angel guidance is to visualize and affirm prosperity in your life right now. Trust that no matter what, everything will be okay. Tap into your manifestation power by focusing on abundance instead of worrying about money as worries only attract money issues. Remember, you get what you think about, whether you want it or not.

Trust that you have everything you need right now. Look past illusions and see the underlying order that is before you. If you need some clarity in your life, spend some time communing with your angels, we are always here supporting you, Always!

Affirmation: "I am growing and expanding in ways that are joyfully balanced."

248

Opportunity to forgive

You have the opportunity to heal, grow, and release negative patterns now.

Angel wisdom suggests that you hold the intention of seeing the inner Divine light and goodness in everyone. The angels can help you release unforgiving thoughts, feelings and energies, and lift you to a higher place of peace and compassion. As you think about your options and possible outcomes, which ones bring the greatest feelings of peace to your body and mind? This is always your answer, the choice is yours. The angels recommend that you choose the path of peace and trust in your choices.

Listen to your heart's truth, there is always a peaceful alternative to conflict within and without. You have grown weary of any negative patterns in your life. To break the cycle, release old toxic thoughts. You can do this by deep breathing, and on each exhalation release your fears, worries, anger and other painful emotions. On your inhale, invite in clear, fresh energy that washes over every cell of your body.

Forgiveness doesn't mean that you are condoning someone's actions; it means that you are no longer willing to carry toxic feelings and thoughts within you. Release, be free, and experience positive patterns through forgiveness of the self first.

Focus on your desires instead of fear or judgments; this includes feelings you have for yourself. Your new peaceful feelings elevate your energy, you then shine like a beacon of light which helps you to attract and manifest what you desire.

Affirmation: "I know that everything happens for my highest good and that my soul is guiding me in everything that I do."

249

You are supported

You have all the power and support of the Universe. You have all that you need to make desired changes in your life right now. Your angel guidance is to visualize and affirm prosperity in your life right now. Trust that no matter what, everything will be okay. Tap into your manifestation power by focusing on abundance instead of worrying about anything. If you are focusing on lack in area of your life, that is what you will attract, if you are focusing on attracting abundance that is what you will attract. Remember, you get what you think about, whether you want it or not.

Trust that you have everything you need right now. Look past illusions and see the underlying order that is before you. If you need some clarity in your life, spend some time communing with your angels, we are always here supporting you, always.

Affirmation: "I am open to receiving what I desire in whatever way or form it appears."

250

Go with the flow

Life is full of change and surprises, move with the currents.

Your guidance is to move with the energy that is surrounding you, for it is in resisting this flow that attracts more of what you don't want and causes more challenges in life.

Ask the angels to assist in opening your mind and your heart to new ideas and fresh options that are in the flow of where you want to go.

There is a solution to every challenge, so look at all things through the eyes of your angels, with love and expectation. Then life force flows freely to and through you. You are supported and surrounded by our love and commitment to your journey. Ask your angels to help you and we are there in an instant.

Bring a new spiritual aspect to all of your relationships. Flow with the love of the Creator and your life will flow freely and with joy.

Affirmation: "I am free and flexible. I bring a spiritual aspect into all my relationships."

251

Switching lanes in life

The changes you have been experiencing are the results of your wanting to open up your heart to more love, to be in your life's mission and consciously be working on your purpose.

Take several deep breaths, and exhale slowly to awaken your energy and to release old patterns that no longer serve you, as it is time to spread your wings and fly. Welcome new opportunities as the old ones are now complete or ready for completion and to let go. Keep your focus on love, service, and spirit. Avoid any naysayers or sceptics, as they just erode your energy, requiring you to work harder at staying centered and balanced.

You are a beautiful being of light. Focus on the beauty within yourself, your kindness, your gifts and your talents and share them with others. Angel wisdom reminds you that whatever you give attention to increases and grows. When you see the beauty within yourself, you see more beauty in your outer world.

Affirmation: "I am love, I am light, I am beautiful. I AM THAT, I AM."

252

Find the moments to celebrate

Look for the joy, the delight and the wonder of each day and rejoice in the gift of it.

Angel wisdom reminds that each day is indeed a gift and so look for the beauty within each experience. Look at each day as an opportunity to understand and heal. In your mind and in your heart, surround yourself, your experiences and anyone involved in a beautiful orb of light. Infuse that orb with loving thoughts. Then, watch as things become more peaceful and balanced. Explore the possibilities of each new day.

Each moment we have with each other is a gift, so spend time with your friends, family and loved ones. Surround yourself with things and people who make you smile and celebrate all things great or small in your life.

Affirmation: "I celebrate each step as it brings me closer to my goals and desires."

253

Dream big

Increase your expectations and see yourself succeeding. Take time today to visualize and dream about your hearts desires. Each day focus on the feelings, and what your dreams will bring to you as if they are already manifested without getting requesting exactly how. Trust that they will come true.

Release any thoughts or feelings of less than, for you are great and powerful. Truly believe that you deserve everything you desire and that you are totally qualified to accomplish anything that you want to. You may feel a bit overwhelmed at times as you move up to a higher plateau in your journey; however you have our reassurance that you are ready. Reach for the stars, know that you are supported and surrounded by love and guidance; all you need to do is ask, then listen to that still, quiet voice within and trust your guidance.

Affirmation:"I deserve all that the Universe has to offer me."

254

Take good care of yourself

Nurture and love yourself as you would your child and loved ones.

Take the time to look at the different aspects of yourself. Ask yourself, "Am I eating food that nourishes my physical temple? Am I breathing fresh air on a regular basis? Is my physical body getting enough movement, and am I taking the time to feed and nourish my spirit as well?"

Your angel guidance is to find foods, activities and inspirations that will assist you in being more connected to your physical self, and the beautiful Mother Earth.

Believe in yourself. Eliminate negative thinking about what nourishes you or how you feel about yourself. Replace any negative thoughts with a desired one such as "I know I can successfully change my eating habits and my life." And, repeat these affirmations at least 5 times a day and watch as your feel more positive and confident about your efforts to adopt a new lifestyle.

Affirmation:"I am committed to keeping myself healthy, whole, and happy."

255

Connecting with the Earth

Send love and light to Mother Earth.

The angels want you to remember that you are spirit with a human mask and an earthly body. When each side is balanced they form a perfect circle, they create a harmonious whole.

Connect yourself with the earth. Walk barefoot on the grass or soil, eat foods from the ground like carrots and potatoes, visit a farmers market in your area, rubbing your bare feet, touching a tree or a plant, or by visualizing roots coming from the bottom of your feet into the earth. Grounding yourself with the earth helps you concentrate and focus, and will also increase your connections with your angels.

Your angel guidance is to connect with Mother Earth and then connect with your angels, forming that perfect circle of life. Do a meditation with us all connected and feel the love, then share that love with others who may not be feeling the strength of this connection.

Affirmation: "I am one with all that is."

256

Hope

Keep hope in your heart.

Remember the Universe wants you to have your heart's desires. There is a limitless pool of which to draw from. Take time out today to clearly decide what you truly want. Then send out positive thoughts and words for the changes that you seek, and fulfillment of your dreams. Ask your angels to help you for we are eagerly at your side guiding and assisting you along the way. You are never alone and we await your next request.

Angel wisdom reminds you it is important to only think about what you desire, not what you fear, as you get what you think about whether you want it or not. Look and be guided by the young ones, for they have much to teach. Watch a child learn to walk and notice how they don't give up, they become more determined to reach their goal. It is inspiring. Use that same determination to create in your own life. It is a power tool that will take you as far as you dare to dream. Dream big dear ones. The joy that is created as you realize your dreams is a powerful tool that assists others who have yet to develop your courage. It is in this way that you assist the growth and evolution of all humanity.

We are here to catch you if you fall. We are here to hold your hand. We are here to love and help you remember your power as you take each step. Keep hope in your heart and trust that tomorrow is a new day, with fresh new opportunities to live in the light.

Affirmation: "I am creating my hopes and my dreams each day."

257

Spiritual growth

Take the time to let your physical body catch up with the new you. During times of great waves of spiritual growth, it is necessary to take time out to rest, relax and rejuvenate. The physical body is the densest of all bodies, and therefore needs more time to catch up with the new you that is emerging. Take the time to rest, nourish and take good care of yourself while you grow, emerge and evolve.

Meditate each day with your guides and angels. Ask for and be open to receiving our support for anything that you need. You can safely move forward knowing that we are with you every step of the way and that you are never alone on this journey. Trust in the signs that we put before you and emerge from your cocoon refreshed with ideas and insights that take you to new heights.

Affirmation: "I trust in the Universe. I grow with love and joy."

258

Celebrate each step

Each step towards health, healing and abundance is cause for celebration. Rejoice for each step that you take leads you to your desired destination and is indeed a cause worth celebrating. It is not always easy to take those first steps toward wholeness and celebrating helps to build the momentum for the step that follows.

Break the cycle of the past and begin anew. Carrying around the past can become a heavy burden and it is time to let that go. Keep only the lessons and the love, and leave everything else behind you. Changing the patterns of the past brings about the blessings you have been asking and praying for. Allow your angels to light the way.

Visualize yourself surrounded by a beautiful clear light of balance and healing. Let your angels guide its colour and intensity, for each day it can be different. Ask your angels to invoke their guidance and help you develop your intuition and inner vision. And remember to trust, offer gratitude, and then celebrate each moment.

Affirmation: "I am happy, healthy and abundant. I am grateful for all that I have."

259

Developing your senses

Meditation is the perfect way to more easily hear and receive our messages.

Come and take a journey with us to a magical land and tap into your inner wisdom and work on expanding your senses. Relax and open your mind to receiving, without directing your thoughts. Just notice the feelings, visions, or ideas that come your way. Call in your entourage of angels to assist you and then be open to the expansion that is taking place.

While you are awake and alert, notice the loving guidance you hear inside your head, or from other people. Notice the feelings that you get and trust in them. If you are unsure, quiet your mind and breath, and ask your heart center to give you more information and then act on the information you receive. Ask your angels to open your third eye and practice using these tools in your everyday life.

Affirmation: "Each day my senses are expanding, opening and becoming more sensitive."

260

Believe in your dreams

Your prayers and expectations have been heard and answered. Your prayers are manifesting. The angels want to remind you to stay positive, and follow the guidance that you are receiving. The angels are working with you every moment that you ask for their assistance, even if you aren't seeing the tangible results yet. Stay on your present path and keep moving towards your goals and dreams.

Oftentimes humans get wary and give up just before they see the results of all their hard work and change course. Your angel guidance is to stick with a plan that feels right in your heart. If you feel something isn't working check in with your guides and angels and from the point of love decide your next step. Be cautious of the advice of others, even the well intentioned, as they don't always see the bigger picture or feel that same connection and all the angles that you can see with your guides. Seek guidance from your angels and trusted advisors and go for it with great gusto.

Affirmation: "I no longer allow doubt, worry or negative pictures in my mind and heart."

261

Setting your intention

Your intentions create your experiences. Take an inventory of your expectations. What do you expect to happen now or in the future? Have you set a plan into motion for where you want to go? Your angel guidance is to consider and evaluate all the options that are before you. Let go of the old and worn out and make room for the new to come into your life. Let go of your head and choose from your heart that which gives you the greatest feelings of joy and feels right.

When you set your intentions, your angels can feel the pure light of your commitment and support you more ways that you can possibly imagine. They can help you replace negative thoughts with more empowering ones, clear the energy that surrounds you and set into motion plans beyond your wildest dreams. Set no limits on what you can achieve and create. Ask for guidance and help and be open to receive the love and wisdom that is available to you.

Affirmation: "I am committed to my vision and choose for my highest good and the good of all; I am open to limitless possibilities in creating my dreams."

262

You are surrounded by support

You've been asking the angels for help with a current situation, your prayers have been heard and we are sending someone from your soul family to help you.

It is time to share your request with others. You've been asking the Universe to send some assistance your way, and indeed we have. Pay attention to the synchronicities, the repeated messages as well as the human with the wise eyes sharing their wisdom. Be patient as you work towards you goal, knowing that doing the journey in a methodical, well thought out fashion, will bring you greater joy along the way. Enjoy each moment of the steps you take.

Angel wisdom reminds you to listen to and for the solutions as you request guidance and assistance. Surround yourself, the situation, the people involved and the entire experience with light and many angels. Be open to the gifts from within and allow yourself to feel peace and serenity. Know that you are surrounded by loving support, both physical and nonphysical beings of love.

Affirmation: "I am supported, loved and powerful. It is safe for me to be fully in my power."

263

Simplify

Simplify your life. This is the perfect time to eliminate clutter from your home, your work life, your heart and your mind. Allow the balance to restore the flow of energy in any aspect that you don't feel is working. Ask yourself what can you immediately shed that will help you achieve this balance once again.

Take some time to see the beauty that surrounds you. Walk on the beach, play with some children in the park, paint a picture, and write your thoughts in a journal. Do something that brings you peace, as this lets you feel joy and helps to clear away any cobwebs that might be hanging around or holding you back.

Take a deep breath and as you returned to center, move forward, even if it is just a little.

Affirmation: "All that I need is within me."

264

Leap of faith

Take that step, and put your heart's true desire into action!

You have set the intention, so now is the time to keep your thoughts, feelings, and actions focused on that target, and you will reach your destination. Trust that you are supported always. Trust that you are worthy and deserving of all that you desire.

Your angel guidance is to awaken the divinity within yourself. Dance, breath, take care of yourself, and always appreciate the beauty that is you. And, go for it.

Affirmation: "I am one with my soul and spirit."

265

Infinite supply

The Universe supplies you with everything you need today, and all of your tomorrows too! There is enough for everyone, there is no need to hurry or force things to happen. Everything is occurring exactly as it should be. Relax and enjoy the journey.

You know what to do. Trust your inner wisdom and take action exactly when the time feels right for you. You are not on anyone's timetable but your own. You might feel an urging in promptings from spirit, as these are often the signs that we send you signalling for you to go forward now. Heed those feelings and trust in them.

Affirmation: "I have the infinite supply of the Universe available to me now."

266

Honour the cycles

Take some quiet time alone to rest, meditate, and contemplate. Learn to read the cycles and how they affect you. Utilize the strength of the moon and how you feel at this time and honour what you need. For many this is a time of retreat and rejuvenation. There has been so much growth and expansion happening that you need to allow your physical body time to catch up. Eat and drink that which nourishes your physical body and take good care of it.

Spend time in meditation and journaling about the messages you receive, the emotions and thoughts that you are having. Be sure to date it. Prepare a ceremony for the full moon and bring out your crystals for recharging. And enjoy the cycles of shedding and rebirth. And get some fresh air today.

Affirmation: "I am growing and expanding in ways that are joyful."

267

Day dream

You will more easily hear and receive our messages if you daydream regularly.

You are a magical person who can manifest your clear intentions into reality. Your daydreams can help you achieve this. We call them conscious journey day dreams. Hold the final outcome of your dreams in your thoughts, the feelings, the joy, the peacefulness that you have at that destination, then while you dreaming, we will offer you guidance on the next best step for you to take, drift off and then listen. There is great power in your ability to create when you visualize the outcome and then listen.

Practice with us each day.

Affirmation: "Each day I am hearing the messages of my guides and angels better and better each day."

268

Contemplating your aspirations

Spend time alone meditating upon that which you desire.

Stretch yourself to fulfill all your potential and hold mighty visions of your desires. The angels guide you to not settle for less than your incredible human spirit can achieve or deserves. Trust that you are supported and that you are worthy of creating your dreams.

As you spend this time of contemplation, you move into a time of greater inner peace and tranquility. Work on developing peace of mind and knowing that you are always provided for. Even if you logical mind cannot currently fathom how this will be achieved.

Angel wisdom reminds you that you can feel serene, even in the midst of great turmoil. You can choose to be happy and peaceful now, no matter what the circumstances.

Affirmation:"I see the love and beauty in everything."

269

See only love

Look past the seeming errors, mistakes and misunderstandings, and see only love. See only love within each person, especially yourself. Your angel guidance is to see yourself through the eyes of your angels and you will see the beauty and love that we see in you. From that point of love, the rest of the world can then be seen from the aspect of unconditional love.

Remember that the human journey is not always an easy one and some people appear to do a 'better' job than others. The angels wish to remind you that you are not all so different, there is no 'more than' or 'less than', all are equal and part of the great Creator energy. Some of you are able to tune into the broader aspect of the experiences more clearly than others.

Remember to send loving thoughts and light around the world to those who might not be feeling it. Call us into your energy field and we can assist in guiding your thoughts to those most tuned to love.

Affirmation: "I offer unconditional love to myself and to others."

270

Notice the signs

Yes, you have been receiving signs. We are sending you signs as answers to your prayers, so look around and notice things that appear three times or more, or, if you think it is a sign, it is. Trust your inner feelings that emanate from your heart. WE are with you, giving you the courage to make the life changes that will help you work on your divine life purpose. WE are with you, supporting you, loving you, helping you.

Use your creative talents to express yourself. This is not limited to painting, drawing, or writing. Each life is carefully orchestrated with you, and your higher self. We are there to help you along the way as you set up the circumstance that will lead you where you want to go, so do pay attention to the signs that lead you, reassure you and support you. Know that we are all working together, even when it feels like you are all alone. You are not alone; you are loved and supported always. We are here, just ask us and we are there. Nothing is too great or too small; we are here to be in service and are eager to be of assistance.

Affirmation: "I easily notice and trust the signs from guides, angels and higher self. I am divinely guided in all ways."

271

Let the transformations take place

To bring in the new you, it is important to cleanse and detoxify your body and your mind and release the old you.

Follow your intuition's guidance about making lifestyle changes. Keep your thoughts and speech positive. Perhaps you have noticed a slump in your energy or perhaps your degrees of joy have been shifting as well. Do not hesitate, even for a moment, to move forward with new habits and patterns. The angels are here to assist you with ideas for cleansing and eating better food and drinks. Avoid harsh chemicals and processed food such as sugar, white flour, etcetera.

Keep your focus on the contents of your mind and the words you speak as these words are the very diet that supports or thwarts you. Choose purity, and we promise you a changed outlook for the better. Open your heart and feel the love we have for you as you emerge from your cocoon to the new spiritual you.

Affirmation: "Each day I am holding loving thoughts for myself, and each thought helps me purify my body, mind and spirit."

272

Ending and beginnings

As the old is released, the new can then enter. Be totally honest with yourself during this process. Look into your heart and you will know the truth within the situations that you are releasing. It is safe and you are supported. WE are here to guide you anytime you ask us for assistance during these changes. Lean upon us for courage, and the strength to take good care of yourself during these times of transitions and growth.

Then, focus only upon your true desires and expect miracles to happen all around you. Dance with the rhythm of life. Take the time to just be in the joy of them moment, even if just for a little while as this helps to clear your energy and bring balance back into your now. Being it the moment of now will help you flow with the cycles of your life.

Affirmation:"I am flowing joyfully with the cycles in my life."

273

Gratitude

When you say thank you to the Universe for its gifts, the energy responds to you with more of that energy.

Angel wisdom reminds you to say thank you for all that you have. Count the blessings for the love, the wisdom, and the guidance you receive as well as for all that you have in the physical realm. Gratitude is the key to opening doors you wish to open, and for closing ones you also wish to close.

There is no need to hurry or to force things to happen. Show your gratitude and trust that everything occurs in perfect timing for you. If you are working at forcing things to happen and they are not, it can be discouraging and then your thought processes go to "it is never going to happen' and then guess what, it is never going to happen. Do you see the block that is up and how you get what you think about whether you want it or not?

Affirmation: "I am grateful for everything in my life." [You can also list some of the things you are grateful for.]

274

Contemplation and understanding

Take some quiet time to rest, meditate and gain understanding of yourself and your current circumstances.

Review your current situations in depth so that you have a clear awareness of the underlying reasons for any challenges or confusion. Become familiar with all aspects, look at the facts and attitudes before you make a decision that becomes your truth.

Self awareness and evaluation are an important foundation in building strong relationships, friendships and work environments. It helps you develop a more balanced way of looking at your world. Invite your angels to help you see the larger pictures and we are gladly there to help you see the others point of view from the vantage of love your angels have for you. This removes judgement and brings in understanding and compassion.

Your angel guidance is go on a retreat or workshop that offers you an opportunity to discover more about yourself, to listen more and talk less, meditate, and surrender any mind chatter and allow your mind to rest, and then from that still point within, gains the understanding.

Affirmation: "I pay attention to and honour my feelings."

275

Follow your dreams

We are leading you toward the answers to your prayers. Please listen to and follow the promptings you feel or hear, as we are communicating to you though your intuition, thoughts, dreams, and meditations. Take time out to relax, get quiet, and get really clear on your desires and dreams so that we are guiding you with clear pictures of your desires. You are surrounded by help on so many levels. Look around and think of who in your circles is best able and willing to help you with your venture and initiate contact.

Notice any repetitious thoughts and feelings, or vivid visions, dreams or auditory messages that you hear in your head or from others or even in songs. These are our loving messages, urging you to take action or make changes. We will make sure that you are safe while you follow your Divine guidance.

See yourself and others through the eyes of the angels, in unconditional love and acceptance.

Affirmation: "My heart is open; I trust in the goodness of the Universe and I am deserving of my share."

276

Receptivity

Allow yourself to receive. This increases your energy and your sensitivities; you are then better able to share yourself and your gifts with others. It is important to always balance your giving and receiving. Often those on the spiritual path naturally care for those in need, it is a part of seeing and feeling more than others, yet this needs to be balanced with receptivity or your flow can diminish or even get blocked. If you feel uncomfortable asking for help, or in receiving the gifts of others, then you are blocking this flow back to you and eventually burn out.

When you receive, you have more resources to give others. Begin by noticing the hundreds of gifts you receive each day, whether it is seeing the beauty of nature, seeing a touching human moment, or being hugged by someone you love. Simply say "thank you" for each gift and know that they are filling up your reservoir of energy and love to share with those in need.

Spend time today just receiving the gifts of Universe.

Affirmation: "I see the gifts of love all around me."

277

Boundaries

Love yourself enough to say no to others demands. Set healthy boundaries on what is acceptable to you and what is not. Set them with love and others will understand and support you.

Angel wisdom reminds you that saying no doesn't mean you don't care or love someone in your life, it means that you know your limits and that it is okay to take time for you, your growth and creating that which you desire. Remember to delegate and also to let things go in love. If this is a challenge for you, invite us into your conversations and we will help you find the right words to say that allows you to express yourself without hurting the feelings of another.

When you are feeling happy, grounded and centered in your own world, you then are better able to be the human angel for those around you. Ask your angels to help you and take that important time out for you.

Affirmation: "I do those things that bring me aliveness."

278

Expect miracles

Trust that your prayers have been heard and are being answered. Trust is the light that illuminates the path before you. Take whatever steps are necessary to keep your mind and your heart filled with faith and trust. Be open to the miracles that surround you. Take note of all that you are grateful for and as you do, more wonderful things happen in your world.

Let go of any worrisome thoughts and keep your thoughts positive. Notice and follow any divine guidance you receive and ask for more as you go along. Engage in a regular spiritual practice, as this will enhance many aspects of your life. Be open to more miracles and more miracles occur.

Affirmation: "My life is filled with miracles"

279

Be flexible

Life is full of changes and surprises. Your angel guidance is to move with the flow of the river of life. Ask your angels to help you open your mind and your heart to new ideas and fresh options. When we accept the idea that there are other alternatives, or see that there is always a bigger picture, new pathways open up before you.

There is always a solution to any situation you have created in your life. Quiet your mind and ask your heart if there is a different path you can take to get where you would like to go if you are feeling stuck. Look at this river you are paddling on with the eyes of love that we have for you and see only the love that surrounds you. The love you share is eternal, just as ours is for you. Explore and enjoy the options and choices that you have and then make your choice. There is no wrong path to take; some are just longer than others. All will eventually get you to where you want to go, so be open and make the choice, then go for it.

Affirmation: "I trust in the flow of the Universe and I am free to flow with it."

280

Laughter

Laughter is the best medicine.

Angel guidance reminds you that when you laugh you release endorphins that make you feel better. Those who are around you when you laugh also release the same endorphins and so the joy and good feelings spread. Get regular doses of laughter each day. Spend some time today finding something to laugh about, someone to laugh with or watch a funny movie or show.

See the humour in your current situations and laugh. When one learns to laugh at themselves and the situations they find themselves in, the answers on how to change things often becomes evident. You release and shake away blocks when you laugh. You feel joyful and hopeful. So, watch a funny movie, watch children play. Do something that makes you laugh each day.

Laughter is a wonderful healer. Let it help you heal. Sometimes a situation cannot heal until you release the challenge completely, so that healing light can enter it. Do not focus on what went wrong, focus on what went right and what is the gift within the situation and know that it is time to let it go.

Do something that makes you laugh, and as you forget and release, your angels can drop in suggestions that let you see things from a different light.

Know that Archangel Michael is always available to offer guidance and protection, invoke him often. Use the power of laughter and friendship in your healing. Laughter is the sunshine that dissolves the darkness, so make merry, and have some fun. And, Laugh often.

Smile and trust that all things get better as you find the peace and harmony within you. Laugh at yourself; laugh with yourself and with others.

Affirmation:"I see the lighter side of life. I love to laugh and laugh often."

281

Love life

You are dearly loved; love each moment, love and live each day of your life.

We know that is not always easy to see the gifts within each moment, and that loving where you are at right now, is sometimes difficult. This is the quickest way we know that can help you on your quest.

Open your heart to all possibilities. Each of you has the ability to transform any situation in your life. Open you tool box of possibilities and let the solutions come forward. There is nothing that has been created that cannot be transformed, it is a universal law. There is no situation in your life that you haven't already planned scenarios of completion. Use the tool of meditation to help you see that there is so much before you.

Trust in your talents and your skills to take you to the next level in all that you do. You are strong and wise and always loved and supported, even if you don't believe it yet. Ask your angels to help you see and feel this, we are here to support you always.

Affirmation: "I recognize and receive all the love the Universe has to offer."

282

Make a commitment

Your prayers and positive expectations are heard and answered. Keep working towards your desires by using focused intent, positive affirmations and paying attention to your inner wisdom.

Angel wisdom reminds you that when you aim for a vision with your full commitment, it must succeed. Your angels work with you, even if you aren't aware of it yet, and we continue to watch over you and everyone involved always. We ask that you take charge. Make the decisions on what you want to do next, don't wait, and take action now. Be clear about the conditions that are acceptable or unacceptable to you. The universe responds when you are clear about your aims and intentions.

Set your intentions today, and then create a plan to keep your focus on what you wish to create. This plan should be done daily as things change as you develop trusting your guidance and therefore plan only the next few steps that get you closer and leave the how's to your angels. Hold the image and feelings of loving the joy and the journey that gets you there. When you find the joy in each step, the end result seems unimportant and you are then living in the now. Keep committed and be in the moment of that always.

Affirmation: "I am committed to my vision."

283

Watch your thoughts

Focused intention is called for at this time. It is important to only think about what you desire, not what you fear. Keep your thoughts, feelings and actions focused and unwavering on getting closer each day to realizing your dreams. This is how you consciously create. Trust, be clear on your desires and watch what you thoughts and words are as you go along. As you learn to master your thoughts, you open the floodgates to abundant creation and then creating is no longer a challenge and you begin to lead that life of magic.

Angel wisdom reminds you to love yourself. Loving others unconditionally is often easier than loving yourself, however it is just as important for you to love and trust yourself, then you find it easier to love and trust the flow of life and unconditional accept all things regardless what the outward appearance may seem. Watch the thoughts and words you use, to yourself, to your life and to others, and transform these to the loving, kind words you use with those you love. Love yourself.

Affirmation: "I choose what thoughts stay in head. Only I am responsible for my focus and intentions."

284

Family

Everyone is family. We are all Family. Our families are our greatest teachers, for these are the ones who love us the most. If you are experiencing any dramas or difficulties within your family, we can assist you in understanding and healing. Your angels wish to remind you that these are the experiences that have the greatest influence on your soul growth and that they are contracts made eons ago.

It is time to emerge beyond what can be seen by the physical or mental body. In your mind and your heart, surround yourself, the people involved and the experience with calming light and many angels. Be open to the gifts within the situations, and allow yourself to feel peace and calmness once again. You can't choose how others react, only how you choose to respond.

You are dearly love and never alone, so invoke our presence anytime you feel you need support, courage and love.

Affirmation: "I am surrounded by love and support always."

285

Gratitude

You are supplied for all of your todays and all of your tomorrows. You have the infinite supply of the Universe available to you, feel how powerful that is and show gratitude for all that you already have. Shower your gifts, and everything truly is a gift, with love. Let golden particles of your love flow forth from your heart into everything that you do, think about, feel, and share. Let it flow into the past, future and present.

Offer a thank you for everyone in your life, no matter what they have brought to you, for each has made you stronger and who you are today. Thank those who have loved and supported you.

And let us, your entourage of helping angels, thank you for being our human messengers.

Affirmation: "I am blessed by this abundant Universe."

286

Easy does it

There is no need to hurry or force things to happen. Everything is occurring in perfect timing and exactly as it should be. The point of the journey is to enjoy the steps along the way.

Angel wisdom reminds you that while a focused intention is important, it does not mean you should not enjoy the process of getting there. It is a fine balancing act, we know. However it is in that balance that you find the joy and harmony that you seek. There is no ONE GRAND plan for each of you, there are many along the road to your next destination, and the balance is in finding the joy on that road, no matter where you are.

Find the gift within each experience and leave no rock unturned as you find that gift. Relax and enjoy this moment, for it won't come again and it is really all that you have.

Affirmation: "I always find the joy in my here and now."

287

Law of Attraction

Think of it not as a reward or a punishment, you have just attracted it, which means you can repel or magnify it as you choose. Angel wisdom reminds you to visualize and affirm only what you desire. Like attracts Like, which means that anything, everyone and everything that you draw into your life is similar to your thought patterns.

If you want to change who or what you attract, hold more positive, loving and joyful thoughts. Your angels are here to help you shift those thoughts. Ask and we are here. If you wish to attract more happiness, think happy thoughts, say happy words and do things that make you happy. This goes for all aspects of your life. You get what you think about, whether you want it or not, therefore as you learn to work with the desired aspects of attraction, you will start attracting more of what you desire.

Affirmation: "I am filled with loving and joyful thoughts."

288

Home

You are here now.

You are already home, just where you are. Find that inner wisdom and create all of the energy of home for you now, here. This is what you are working towards, creating heaven on earth, and you have all the means within you to create just that now.

If you wish to create a healthy change within your home, begin by looking into your heart and see the truth that dwells there. Begin by doing little things that create more harmony for you, and as you create more harmony, you create an opportunity for others to create harmony in their own lives. Know that we are always here to support you with words, and ideas to help you on the way. Transformations will take place as you look in your heart and change what you would like to change within yourself. As you change within, the world changes around you. It is therefore for the good of all for you to find that within yourself. How refreshing.

Then create a peaceful environment around you. Get rid of things that you don't like, regardless of where they came from. Surround yourself with things that have meaning and that you love. This is creating a new space and energy in your physical surroundings. Do you see how as one changes, the others change and it ripples out. Others will feel the change in the energy and join in the flow that is created. Create the energy of home all around you and you will begin to see it others.

Affirmation: "Home is where my heart is and it is always with me."

289

Relationships

Cultivate your primary relationship, which is with yourself.

The most important relationship you will ever have is with yourself, every other relationship follows from there. To attract, heal, or balance a relationship, balance or heal this within yourself. As this begins to happen, your outward relationships will also blossom and change.

Your angels want you to know that they are here to help you always. We can bring a human angel to you if you ask for assistance, we ask that you pay attention to the signs we put before you. Call upon Archangel Michael if you need to feel more strength, courage, confident, or removing lower thoughts or energies from around you.

Affirmation: "I am strong, confident and protected."

290

Synchronicity

Your prayers and questions are being answered by synchronistic events. Notice them in order to increase their flow. You are receiving wonderful ideas as answers to your prayers. They are real indeed and most trustworthy as they are coming from us through you. You can safely move forward knowing that we, your angels are with you every step of the way, supporting you, and lighting the path that is before you.

The more you notice these signs, the more signs come your way. So take the time to tap into us and all that we have to offer and share with you and notice the answers and assistance that is coming your way. Make it fun and make it a joyful part of your day. We love to see and feel joy and love and it is a strong manifesting energy.

Affirmation: "I notice the signs that show me I am on the best path and eagerly act upon them."

291

Trust

Trust in yourself. Trust that you do indeed deserve it all. This is one of the most difficult tasks many of you face each day.

Sometimes when humans have trusted, they felt they were let down, first by others and then by themselves. The angels wish to remind you to begin again fresh and new. If you are holding on to past experiences and old results, you will get more of the same. That is the universal law of attraction. It is therefore important for you to focus on what is happening now and is before you in the present moment, and not keep looking back to the past.

First, put your faith in yourself. Listen to your intuition; listen to the emotions that come from your heart. Release any of the energy of the mental body, the ego, as this often stops you from moving forward or seeing the results that you desire. Ask us to help you lose any fears that might be blocking you from enjoying unconditional trust in yourself and the Universe.

Let your angels flood you with our love and allow it to flow into your heart and your mind. Clear old thought patterns and we can help you to release them. Allow yourself to spontaneously feel that love and trust that you are powerful and deserving.

Affirmation: "I have all the resources I need to create my desires; I trust in the abundant, infinite Universe."

292

Surrender

Whatever you resist in life persists.

Ask your angels to help you dissolve all the resistances in your life. Clear away inner conflict and struggles, the rigid mindsets and habits so that they can flood your life with higher truths and with joy.

When you surrender to the guidance of your higher self, all the energy that you have been using up in resistance is now free to be used in creating other things such as inner peace, harmony and most of all love.

Let go of any old guilt, remember that you are a most perfect child of creator energy, and just as you are that spark, as are all those in your life. See only the love that we have for you, for each other, see only love.

Affirmation: "I surrender to the flow of life."

293

Focus upon your strengths

View yourself with compassion and love, always.

Anytime you find yourself thinking or feeling poorly about yourself, focus upon your strengths instead. Use daily positive affirmations to lift your energy and faith. Your strengths include your loving heart, pure intentions, talents and skills, all of those aspects of growth that you have been working on. The more you honour and bless your strengths and assets, the stronger they become.

Be flexible and know that life is full of changes and surprises. Keep your mind and heart open to new ideas and fresh options. There is always a solution to every situation, so look at all things with eyes of love and expectation. Then life force will flow freely through you and to you.

Affirmation: "I realize that all things I thought were wrong with me are gateways for me to discover my greatest strengths."

294

Health and healing

It is time for the healing within the 'family' to begin in a new way. It is time for an emotional experience within a family unit; this can be a soul family, DNA family, a work family. They are a unit of close bond whether everyone is aware of it or not. It is time to call upon your guides and angels to assist in understanding and healing this group. In your heart and in your mind, surround everyone involved in this family unit with a calming blue light and call in all of your angels to assist in sharing love or for health and healing.

Picture everything healed. See the celebration in the healing and the bond that it creates and hold that image until it materializes in the physical realm. Just as you are evolving to a higher state of being, so are all of your family, friends and life situations.

Affirmation: "I feel peace within myself and this situation." [List the healed situation].

295

What do you aspire

It is time to set your sights on what you truly desire.

It is time to let go of the old and worn out so that the new can come in. It is time to stretch yourself to fulfill all your potential and to hold mighty visions indeed. The angels guide you to never settle for less than you desire, and know that you can achieve anything you set your heart to. Dream big and let no one diminish you.

Give your cares and worries to us angels, and allow us to take your challenges and work with them with you. Ask us for help, we will guide and inspire you to raise your vibration and consciousness to another level.

Let your spirit soar and aim high indeed.

Affirmation: "I do those things that evolve, inspire, and uplift myself."

296

Beginnings

Life is a series of cycles and a time of rebirth is indicated now.

Be persistent in your pursuit of your desires. Use action and positive thinking to make your dreams manifest into form. Do not be afraid to let go of the familiar, for the new cannot enter until the old and outworn have departed.

This can mean a new phase in your current relationships, new relationships, fresh new ideas or the development of qualities in you like laughter, light and hope. It may bring about a complete change in life as you know it. Trust that everything will be handled in a fair and just manner for the good of all, which also includes you also.

Your angel guidance is to accept the new, celebrate each step along the way and congratulate yourself often as this signifies the growth process is happening.

Affirmation: "I welcome and nurture the new in my life."

297

Take time to play today

The angels say that it is important to play.

Playing creates joy, which creates miracles and manifestation. When you play, it creates a wondrous fresh energy around you that is perfect for new ideas and solutions to come bubbling forth. We can more easily get our messages and inspirations through to your thoughts as all the 'other' thoughts that often block you from hearing our messages are out of the way.

Trust in the divine guidance you tap into after you have been playing about with no agenda. Just relax in the grass and look up at the sky, see the sun, see the clouds, take a deep breath and then let our messages flow to you and through you. Enjoy the energy, recall it often and let it help you manifest each day.

Go outside and play today!

Affirmation: "I take time and space for myself to be in the moment and feel joy all around me."

298

Intentions

Stay focused upon your intentions, desires, and priorities. Pay attention to the doors that are opening, and learn from the doors that are closed.

Keep a positive outlook about your dreams, and imagine that they've already manifested into reality. Spend time each day devoted to projects that are dear to your heart.

If you are stuck or indecisive, the Universe doesn't know what you want. It is important to clearly decide what direction or goals you choose and focus on them, and then the energy created is stronger.

If you are unsure what the next step on your path is, ask the angels. We will help to guide you. It is your responsibility to take the steps through those doors you choose take. Know that everything works within the Universal Laws, such as the Law of Attraction and the Law of Divine Timing. This means that the vibration you are putting out is what you receive, and that certain pieces of the puzzle must be in place so that other parts can come into play. If you skip, rush or ignore certain pieces or parts, the plan lacks a solid foundation, and you don't see the results you desire.

Decisiveness is the catalyst for the angels to clear the way for your manifestations. Let go of the fears or the worries and focus only on the destination you intend to reach. Enjoy the journey along the way.

Affirmation: "I am always in the perfect place at the perfect time."

299

Explore your options

This is a good time to make changes in your life.

It is a good time to look at other possibilities that are before you. Have faith that within you is the power to manifest anything that you can imagine creating in your life. It is important as you are exploring to remain positive and focused as well as to follow the guidance that you are receiving for us as we surround you with help when you ask. Sometime this help comes in ways that you wouldn't have come up with on your own, trust us and trust in yourself to have all the powers that are necessary to take you to another level.

You and your loved ones are protected and safe. WE are surrounding you with love as you start to feel this new level of trust that is necessary to take things to a higher vibration.

Affirmation: "I am open to new ideas and am safe to explore them."

300

Pay attention to the signs

Notice the repetitious signs and your inner guidance.

There is much wisdom in the signs we put before you. When you notice more of these answers to your prayers it is as if the Universe then gives you more. Actually they were always there; it is just that you did not notice them before. As you expand your light and understanding more is available for you to utilize. More opportunities, more love, more abundance, the list is endless just as you are.

Angel wisdom reminds you that you have only just begun to tap into that which has always been available to the seekers. You are just getting started, so have patience with yourself and the process and do not give up.

Affirmation: "I notice the messages from my guides and angels more and more each day and I am so grateful."

301

Hope

Please do not worry. Everything is going to be fine and the future ahead of you looks bright.

The angels wish to remind you that the Universe wants you to have your heart's desires. It is simply waiting for you to believe you deserve it. It truly is a kind Universe and everyone within it is working in your favour, even if it doesn't always feel that way. There are really no tests, blocks or obstacles in your way, except your own projections of fear and failure into your future.

Take a moment and quiet your mind. Feel your angels caress

as they encircle you with new energy of trust, hope, and optimism, and let these energies fuel your today's and tomorrow's. Ask your angels for help and they will fan the sparks of potential and bring them to life.

Affirmation: "I hold positive thoughts and intentions for my todays and tomorrows and know that all of my expectations are fulfilled."

302

Find the blessings

What appears to have been a loss, needed to fall away.

The angels wish to remind you to look around and recognize the blessing in the midst of apparent challenges. What appears to be a problem is actually part of the answer to your asking. Trust that you are safe and protected and trust in the infinite wisdom within you to see the blessings that surround you.

Take a look around and notice that your outer world reflects your inner world. Are there simple changes you can make that will then be reflected all around you? As you seek the blessings and the beauty in all things around you, things in your outer world and shifts in your thought processes change and watch as each one shifts to a new vibration as they are truly interconnected. You will feel healthier and more alive and feel the life force flow freely through you.

Affirmation: "I easily see the gifts in all that I do."

303

Spiritual wisdom

Wisdom is listening to the Divine promptings within you.

Your angel guidance is to connect to that still, quiet center and listen to the wisdom of your soul. We bring to you esoteric information and symbols, and assist you in understanding and working with spiritual truths. As you develop and trust your inner wisdom, life takes on a new perspective. Dramas and fears become insignificant in comparison to the magnificence of the big picture, the love and sheer beauty that can be felt.

See the beauty within each sunset in your life and trust that the sun will rise again on all of your tomorrows. It is time to embark on the next part of your journey in the light of the new expanded you that is emerging. Know that we are with you through every phase and cycle.

Affirmation: "I listen to my inner wisdom."

304

You are powerful

It is time to realize your true power and that it is safe to be empowered.

You are born with a natural power that often gets stifled or dialled down, and now is the time to bring forth this strength that lies within you. Stretch yourself to fulfill all of your potential and hold mighty visions for yourself. You are surrounded by magical energy and opportunities. Find the wisdom within you which enables you to heal, grow and release any undesired patterns. Hold the intention of seeing and feeling your inner Divine light and goodness and then see it in others.

We will help you release any unforgiving thoughts, feelings, and energies, and lift you to a higher place of compassion and peace. Ask for help from the angels and they will guide and inspire you to raise your consciousness and live at a higher level. Nurture that powerful strength within you that has always existed and supported you.

Affirmation: "I have the strength and resources that I need, always."

305

Truth

Live your truth with integrity.

For these two actions lead to the serenity that is so desired. The angels suggest that now is the time to take action towards being in your truth. Begin to live your life from your truth, no one else's. And worry not about how they live their life; focus your attention on your life and what you want to create for yourself. Worry not how others see you, for that is their issue. We are not saying to ignore others; we are saying to love each other just as you are, regardless. Honour them for the choices they make in their journey, regardless if you would do it differently. Honour yourself for the choices you have made, even if it seems you might have gone off the path at times. It is those side journeys that assist your growth and expansion, and helps you gain great insight and clarity as you go on your path.

There is no 'one path' for anyone. There are choices and different routes to take along the way. Look where you are at today and be thankful for all that led you this place, regardless! Acceptance means unconditional love. Accept everyone exactly as they are, without judging, blaming or wanting to change them, this includes you as well.

Live in your truth with integrity, trust the wisdom of your heart and lovingly go forward.

Affirmation: "I will always endeavour to be my authentic, hearts centered self and harmonize my desires with those of my soul."

306

Intentions

Your intentions create your experiences.

What do you intend to happen? Where are your current thoughts, as your thoughts and your feelings about that which you desire mirror what happens next. Whatever you expect to happen are the seeds of your intention. Your angel guidance is to choose and infuse your intentions. See yourself and others as balanced, peaceful and successful. Open your heart to love, your mind to your inner wisdom, and follow your path to the happy outcomes you desire.

Dream big! Your dreams are coming through in ways you might not possibly think of. Be open, be positive and know that you are supported by your angels and your guides. Keep going, no matter how things might seem around you; know that it will bring you to a higher place. As you begin to feel hope and support, others will feel it in your aura and it helps them in numerous ways.

Affirmation: "I am happy, healthy and abundant."

307

Energize with water

Spend some time near water, such as a lake, river, or the ocean. If you cannot physically go to the water, then take a spirit journey in your meditation and allow the spirit of the water to cleanse and revitalize you.

This will recharge and energize you. Drink plenty of fresh clean or filtered water, as this too will recharge and energize you. Water offers wonderful cleansing benefits, outside and inside of your beautiful physical vessels, which are made up of mostly water. Water is a conductor and allows for the angels to connect with the humans in a stronger way, it amplifies our messages.

Surround yourself with positive people and situations, avoid negativity. Water can wash away sadness, pain, and the energy of others. Engage in purification meditations involving water often, whether it is a soaking in a bath filled with sea salts and special oils and candle light, or a swim in a freshwater stream, you're sure to feel the difference that water makes in your life.

Affirmation: "I welcome the properties of water to cleanse my energy and body."

308

Positive energy

You are sensitive to the energy that surrounds you.

Angel wisdom recommends that you go on a negativity diet at this time. This means avoiding negative or harsh influences, both internally and externally at this time. Avoid negative discussions with yourself and others. Avoid pessimistic programs, people and things. Avoid foods that are processed and loaded with chemicals (if you can't pronounce it, you shouldn't eat it). This allows for you to cleanse yourself and work through hidden blocks that could slow you down, slowing down the manifestation process.

Spend some time working with the energy in your home or office, apply some basic principles of feng shui and let the energy around you flow more freely. Give away items that you don't absolutely love, as this frees up energy to bring in the things and opportunities that you desire. Bring the energy of Joy into your surroundings, this allows you to attract and create your present and future moments in a higher light.

Affirmation: "I am surrounded by positive energy and joy at all times."

309

Enjoy the outcome

Take time to savour the moments. As you look back and reflect upon all that you have accomplished, reward yourself. Take a time out and go for a walk in the beauty of Mother Nature, get a massage, go for a coffee with an old or new friend.

Do something for yourself today that makes you feel special and alive. Enjoy those moments of victory, no matter how small they may be. All steps are worthy of a celebration.

Change is always happening; it is part of the cycle of life. Bringing in the changes you dream about in your heart is the key to a more joyous journey. Keep you focus on your desires, live in your truth and follow your passion. Do your best, always, and everything will fall into place. Change signifies that your journey is evolving and that is after all what you came to earth to experience.

Affirmation: "My world is filled with love, joy, beauty, peace and wonder, always."

310

Clarity

Where are your thoughts? It is important in these times of shorter 'lag time' in your manifestations that you be clear on what the focus of your thoughts are.

Take some time to sit quietly so you can find the stillness within. Then you can shine a pure, clear light into every area of your life. Look at what makes you happy, what brings you joy, ask us to join with you and we can help to light the way to a new way of seeing, a new way of being. Get really clear on what it is you are actually thinking about.

Perhaps you need a little more help at first, to see what the vibration of your thought processes are. Take a class or see a spiritual counsellor that assists you in your evolution, to empower your path. There is much wisdom available to assist in the transformations, trust your heart. Trust that deep, wise, still place within you, always.

Affirmation: "I create quiet time to receive the guidance and clarity that I need."

311

Fully supported

We hear your prayers for assistance and support.

Ask your angels to help you heal your thoughts and emotions.

This assists in removing any blocks that stand between you and all that you desire to create. Open your heart to receiving. As you honour and follow the guidance of your heart, the more prosperity and abundance comes your way.

Look at your belief systems about where you feel that you are blocked. Can you see where this was created? We are always with you to help and assist; this is why you came to do this journey with guardian angels by your side, so you would know that you are never alone and always supported. Just ask and we will go to work on your behalf, always, even if you don't feel it, trust that we are there.

The more you release control and trust, the more ideas, thoughts, feelings and knowingness will flow to you and through you.

Affirmation: "I am supported, I trust in the abundance of the Universe. I am deserving of all that I desire."

312

Be true to yourself

It is time for you to make your real feelings and beliefs known. Share the beauty of who you are with yourself and others. Let people see your true nature. Let people feel your wisdom, and follow your heart.

Yes, your relationships will change when you 'come out of the closet'. Ones that aren't evolving will naturally drop away, and others will deepen because you will know that you are loved and respected for who you truly are. This is very freeing to your soul.

Trust and follow your intuition. You are being divinely guided right now. Trust the knowingness, the visions, or the inner voice that are trying to share with you to enhance your journey. Know that you are spiritual supported in this process by the guides and the angels.

Use positive affirmations each morning to assist you in all that you wish to manifest. This is a powerful tool if you choose to use it. Before or immediately after arising, spend a few minutes thinking about your desires. Allow yourself to imagine that they've already manifested. Set your intention for what you would like to create in your day today (each day). And as you go about your day, let go of any judgments about yourself or others. Speak your truth with **LOVE**. Allow others to get to know the real you.

Trust your authentic self, the more authentic you are, the higher the energy and success of all of your projects.

Affirmation: "I am true to myself; my life is growing better each day."

313

Balancing your masculine energy

It is time to bring the masculine energy into balance within you.

Sometimes there is a need to heal a 'male' energy relationship first, then moving on to that balance within. Your outer world represents your inner world, so take a look around and see if you notice an imbalance of the ego, father energy, or actual father. Take a look at those relationships that have residual energy left unhealed and allow them heal.

Angel wisdom reminds you to be open hearted, with yourself and others. We applaud you for the courage to take down all the walls and expose your humanness. Ask your angels to help you dissolve any masks or barriers so that your beautiful new self can emerge like a butterfly from its cocoon.

Affirmation: "My choices and opportunities are expanding each day."

314

Healing a broken heart

The Heart must heal. It is time to let go of a past hurt, betrayal, grief, loneliness, anger or any other mental or emotional feelings. Let go of the past so that there is room for the new to enter. Angel wisdom reminds you that the love that you send out into the world is an important part of your life purpose, and also what you receive back.

This can take some time so be patient with yourself. Treat yourself as you would any ailing person, with caution, gentleness, and tenderness. Next, get out into the world, not in a harsh fashion, go for walks in the park, the forest, the mountains, by a stream or the ocean, anywhere that lightens your mood and outlook, and fills you with fresh oxygenated air. Spend some time with our great healer, mother earth and regain your foothold on the planet. Your heart will mend and you are ready to dance among the living once again.

Affirmation: "Love is eternal, regardless of where I am."

315

Get quiet

Spend time with us and with nature.

This is a time to get clear on who you are and where you want to go next. Take a walk near the ocean, or in a forest, be with the plants and the trees. Let them clear the energy fields around you and let them assist in your healing. Take deep breaths of their gifts and share yours with them, feel the love exchanged in the experience then sit down and look at where you are, decide what should stay and what should go. What is your next choice, what is the next step you want to take on that path?

Strengthen and nurture your relationships with your guides and angels. There is a group of us waiting to work with every one of you. Allow us to enter your dreams and your life. Let us help to guide the way. Invite us in (we promise to behave) and always remember, we come in love and we are always governed by free will.

Affirmation: "The clearer my desire, the more clear is the path before me."

316

Bringing creativity in to your new beginnings

To create prosperity, explore you creative potential now.

Creativity is energy for adventure and change. It can mean a new phase in a relationship, germination of a new idea, and inspiration with an old idea, developing qualities like laughter, light and hope. Let your imagination flow. If you do not know how to channel the force, you may feel restless or dispirited. This is a sign to seek out something more.

So, ask your angels to help you to direct your creative energy toward something worthwhile, except the new when it arrives, and trust that your material needs are provided for. Trust your intuition and inner guidance to manifest your dreams into reality. You live in an abundant universe and there is enough of everything for everyone. When you understand this principle you free up much of your energy for your creative pursuits.

Affirmation: "I enjoy my creative powers and use them for the highest good. I trust in the infinite Universe."

317

Life purpose

Part of your life purpose, meaning this physical life, is to evolve and experience. This means there are always going to be beginning and endings. Always the cycle of life continues. The trick in being a master is in managing to create a more harmonious flow instead of huge waves and then droughts.

Right now is the time to let go of the old, that which no longer serves your highest good, be it your thoughts, things or emotions. Release that which you no longer require or need to make way for the new opportunities of abundance. Allow nice even waves of prosperity to wash in, thus assisting with the flow of your purpose for life.

Worry not about what your life purpose, for this changes as you change. Spend your energy and focus on creating an environment that brings peace, love, harmony and cooperation with others. Follow your heart and your passions in life and you will be living a life with purpose.

Affirmation: "My life purpose illuminates me and shows me the way."

318

Stay optimistic

Keep your thoughts positive

Your dreams will come true if you keep your focus, drive and determination focused on the final outcome. Fear not that it will mean an ending, as it will signify new beginnings in undreamed of ways. Ask your angels for direction and guidance as well as to buoy your courage and trust. We are always willing to be your angelic assistants. Then, pay attention to your feelings and thoughts as these are often signs to show you the way. Learning to sense your feelings about situations is the best guide available to you and is always a part of you.

Transmute any lower or stagnant energy into something that feeds you. Use the violet flame of purification to turn anything you desire into positive, productive energy that can be utilized right now to strengthen and feed you, the earth and everything.

Keep tolerance and forgiveness in your heart always and walk the path of light with us each day. Your angel guidance is to remember that a sense of humour and optimism will take you far indeed.

Affirmation: "I know many good things are coming my way."

319

Manifestations

Your desired aspirations are now available. This is the process by which all thoughts transform into tangible form. What do you desire to create right now?

This is the time to take real control of consciously creating in your life. If things look bleak, this is the time to turn the energy around. First look at where your thoughts are. Thoughts are transformed into tangible things; everything begins as an idea, then the idea meets with a feeling. If the feeling is loving and nurturing, the idea and the feeling create the embryo of the manifestation.

Things are going to change, the question is, which direction are they changing? Rethink what you're going to do next. Meditate, keep calm, and take what action you can. Take good care of your health. Start reading, take time out for yourself, and turn your face to the sun. Take a walk in the woods, enjoy your loved ones, your food, and care for your health. Life is complex, yet so simple.

Angel wisdom reminds you that your intention into this new stage is a most important step and the universe's abundance is open to you. There may be a new beginning of some kind, and new challenges and opportunities are definitely on the horizon. You are about to start another phase in your karmic journey.

A brilliant new phase of this grand adventure called YOUR LIFE is about to enfold, embrace it with passion.

Affirmation: "I allow the abundance of the Universe to manifest through me now."

320

Change happens

Take some time to rest, recover and retreat from everything if you are not clear on the next step.

You've dreamed for change, and now it is coming. With this change come some major decisions that can be life altering and not always the easiest ones to make. There are many choices and paths that can lead you where you want to go. All paths will eventually lead you where you want to go, some are just shorter or less eventful than others.

How do you want to enter into this time of change? Clearly we hope. Your Angel guidance is to take time to get really clear. Do a review and complete the unfinished tasks, get them done and take a time out from other worldly activities while you do this as much as you possibly can. Use this time to meditate and clear your physical world, emotional world and your mental world. Get them into order and balance so that you can have all the energy you desire to focus on the shifts happening in your spiritual realm as well.

Make the time for a daily spiritual practice of meditation, everyday.

Affirmation: "I am blessed. My life is growing better each day."

321

Meditation and contemplation

It is time to create a clear vision of what it is you truly want. Where is it that you choose to go? What lies within your heart? It is these thoughts and dreams that you should be focusing all of your energy towards.

Create the picture, create the movie of what it is you want and be totally clear. Then begin to focus on the streams that will take you there **now**. What can you do **Now,** that will get you one step closer to that which you desire?

You are surrounded by support on so many levels. There are people around you and there are people who will feel your shifting vibration and be drawn to you. There are your guides and your angels who are always ready and willing to work with you side by side to help you create in the physical realm, just ask.

Relax, Enjoy wherever it may be that you find yourself this day. Trust that you can make the best possible day, no matter what is happening around you, and see the beauty and gift in all that is.

Affirmation: "All that I need is within me. I am living my greatest potential each day."

322

Creating sacred spaces

Angel wisdom suggests that creating sacred spaces wherever you are is important.

Everywhere you are is a sacred space. Creating sacred space assists in keeping yourself in balance and connected to Mother Earth, and feeling the unconditional love that can be shared.

Begin by creating sacred space in your home. Create an alter, or a room for creating ceremony, clear away clutter and things you don't absolutely love. Begin creating sacred space in your workspace, clear clutter, remove everything you don't love that can be removed, and make things you can't move appealing. Start with little things and watch as your space transforms and then things around it begin to transform. Say a little prayer creating sacred space around you as you go about your chores and mixing with the energy of others.

Each one of you is sacred, and each one of you is revered. We wish that you could feel our love and admiration for you at every moment, some of you can feel it right now, for some of you it will come. As you begin to feel our love, begin to see and feel the love that connects each one of you to the other.

Affirmation: "Everywhere I go, I am surrounded by sacred space and I am filled with peace, love, and harmony."

323

Detach from drama

View life as a movie that you know will have a happy ending, or at the very least, an ending that is resolved with the best, highest possible outcome. Have compassion for everyone and everything, yet do not get pulled into the energy of the drama or let it pull you down in any way. As you begin to focus on the positive, you will attract a positive resolution for all concerned.

Let go of attempts to make everyone happy. Allow others to make their own choices in life. Focus your energy on choices for you. When you are positive, you keep directing a stream of high vibrating energy with your thoughts, words and deeds. You choose your thoughts and attitudes, so focus on loving, abundant and successful outcomes in every area of your life.

Affirmation: "I am positive and strong."

324

Understanding yourself

Self awareness is the foundation on which to build as you explore who you really are. From self awareness we build healthy, strong relationships, friendships and work relationships. Understanding your personality is a basis for understanding your spiritual self, your emotional self and your physical self. It helps you to understand why you chose to do an earth journey. We are honoured to assist you with this.

Your angel guidance is to examine yourself and your current life circumstances in depth so that you have a clear awareness of the underlying reasons for any situation you are not completely satisfied with. Understand your attitudes and feelings and why you are not satisfied and what you need to be satisfied, and then make your next choice. As you gain a greater understanding of yourself and your choices, you see a greater picture in play in everyone's lives, including your own.

Affirmation: "I seek understanding of myself and my life."

This is truly the most important relationship you have, the one between you and you.

325

Celebrate your progress

The angels say that today is about celebrating who you are and how far you have come. Take some time to celebrate who you are and the transformations and expansions you have made on your journey. It isn't always an easy task to be in a human process, yet the joy, rewards, and expansion that you have experienced as a soul has been astounding.

Look into your heart and see that you have come through many tests and trials and there were many times you felt you might not make it out of the forest, feeling there are so many obstacles, that it just isn't worth the journey. Yet at other times you have created magnificently, and felt so much love and joy. Lean upon us if you need courage and strength. Trust that you have indeed made tremendous progress and that each day is better than the one before.

Your angel guidance is to celebrate today, and celebrate all that you have and do. Focus on the joy of today and trust that you can tackle tomorrow in a new light.

Affirmation:"I am joy filled, and love to explore the wonders of life."

326

Empowerment

You're more powerful than you realize. It's safe for you to be powerful!

You inner power wants to surface. Your connection with the divine has become powerful. During this time you are often filled with many different feelings, confusion, excitement, fear, and wonder. You want to be totally immersed in your spiritual life and studies, wishing you could read, study, learn, meditate, and do healings on a full time basis.

For some of you this may be possible. Be sure to keep your focus and your thoughts on what you are creating. Trust that you are supported, loved, and guided at each moment. Don't worry about how your future will blend with your spiritual growth, just trust that it will.

Angel wisdom reminds you that if your focus is on, "What impact will my new spiritual pursuits have on my job, marriage, or friendships? These worries create a fear that may erode the enjoyment your spiritual studies bring you. Surrender those feelings, as what you resist in life persists. Ask you angels to help you dissolve all the resistances of your ego (the inner conflict and struggle) so that we can help flood your life with higher truth and joy.

Begin taking small steps towards your goals of spiritual growth and understanding. Begin to focus on the service you can offer humankind at this stage in our evolution. Find ways that allow you to practice your growth and share your knowledge that allows you to be in your truth now, and to continue on your current path of growth and empowerment. As you begin to swim in the stream of your desires, on joyful service, you begin to feel that this stream continues to support your growth, and you begin to enjoy the shifts you see around you.

Use your power, talents, passions and interests to make the world a better place, put your focus on giving and receiving, then through the Law of Attraction, you'll receive all of the support you'll need.

Affirmation: "Everything I do is something I want to do and brings me all that I need to live out and fulfill my life purpose."

327

Crystal clear intentions

Be crystal clear about what it is you desires and intentions. Focus upon what you truly desire with unwavering trust and conviction. It is important to get yourself completely clear on what you desire to create in your world. The more clear you become, the stronger the vibration that you put out to the universe, the more determined and focused your path becomes and therefore the clearer the path that is before you. When you are undecided in your thoughts, then that is the vibration that is emanating from you, and that is what you see happening before you. If you are not getting the results you want or the satisfaction and joy that you know are your birthright, take a look at what you are expecting to receive. Ask yourself where your mind set is at?

Your angel guidance is to use the power of desired affirmations. Make a commitment to do them regularly and with all of your hearts conviction, then you will see more tangible results created in your physical realm, as if by magic. Don't over analyze it or let doubt stray into your thoughts. Cancel or transmute them as soon as you realize your thoughts are less than you desire. Trust in your ability to create. Ask for assistance from your guides and angels, and most importantly, get really clear about what you want and then, enjoy the journey.

Affirmation: "I am focused and getting more clear each day about my path and purpose."

328

Let your spirit soar

Awaken the God/Goddess within you. It is time to let the real spirit *You* emerge.

Release him/her and let them soar to their true magnificence. Have faith, and trust that being who you truly are, will feel so freeing. You become more joyful, peaceful and happy when you can be your true self. Yes, there are things that might change in your world, as your new vibration won't always match those that you love or have in your life right now, however just love them anyway, let them go, and know that they too are on their path, whatever that may be for them.

Take some quiet time to meditate and connect with the divinity within you. See the divinity in others and all things around you. Remain focused and positive, and follow your guidance. As you bring forth the true you, you become aware that you are always connected with us and it is an instantaneous connection. We are a part of each other. Feel our love emanate from inside of you. Let it flow. Let it surround you and feel the support that you have. Know that you are never ever alone and always, always, always deeply loved.

Affirmation: "I love you enough to accept you for who you are; I love you unconditionally."

329

Be the magician in your life

You are a magical person who can manifest your clear intentions into reality.

Open your heart. Trust in your ability to clearly go forward with your dreams and intentions. The only obstacle in your way is the mental energy that surrounds you. What you believe you will get and or what you deserve. This includes and comes from the ego.

Be sure that you don't allow the admiration and thoughts of others for your part in this journey to go to your head. Just as you are magical, so are they, and as you begin to see that beauty in others, your life will begin to shift and change. Be in the moment of it and then release it and continue forward.

Your angel guidance is to spend time setting your priorities, and grounding yourself regularly. Connect with your Earth. Feel her love and emanate it to others. Live your life by example and for yourself and the growth of your soul. Your angels want you to know how loved and supported you are and that you are never alone and we so admire your courage and strength as you become your magical self while in the limits of physicality.

Affirmation: "I am infinitely abundant and magical."

330

Be honest with yourself

Be true to yourself in all of your activities and action.

Let go of anything in your life that is inauthentic, and let all your actions mirror your highest intentions and values. If something in your life is not working, it is time to release it and let it go. Cut the cords completely with Archangel Michael's sword of truth, which is available to all those who ask for it. It may be that you still have some unfinished business, so ask your angels to help you better understand why you chose this project and how you can complete it and let it go.

You are making steady progress, even though it doesn't always seem so. Trust that you are supported and let the divine light of love transform any troubling conditions. Angel wisdom reminds you to be thankful for all that you have the tangible and intangible.

Your angel guidance is to count your blessings. When you offer gratitude to the Universe, it responds generously to you. Gratitude is the key to opening the doors of abundance.

Affirmation: "I am grateful for everything in my life."

331

You are safe

You are safe and spiritually protected at all times.

All your needs are being met and always will be. Release any tension or worry, as it blocks you from your sacred mission of sharing your light and your love with others. Instead, the gentle essence of a joyful heart and laughter will set your power into motion. Ask yourself why you have any tension in your mind or body unless you believe that somehow you or your loved ones are unsafe? And how could you be unsafe when you can call upon your entourage of spiritual warriors to watch over and assist you? Trust that the angels are watching over you and your family when you remember to invoke us.

It is safe for you to move forward and act on your inspirations. It is time to take your ideas to the next level and manifest them into physicality. Quiet your mind and listen to the gentle reassurance that everything has been taken care of. Stay in a quiet and receptive state, without worrying exactly how your desires will manifest. Trust that it is safe to move forward and begin taking the next step.

Affirmation: "It is safe for me to be powerful. I am safe and protected, always."

332

You have Divine knowledge

It is time to share your Divine wisdom with others.

Humans learn and teach best by example. The angels want to remind you that this cycle of leading by example are your strongest attributes in teaching others about spirituality and leading a spiritual life.

Your angel guidance is to connect with your inner wisdom by quieting your mind and body, and when you are relaxed and in a receptive vibration, listen to that still, quiet voice that emanates from your heart. Trust your connection to this infinite wisdom that every being has access to. As you make this spiritual practice a part of your everyday life, you feel more balanced and serene, regardless of what is occurring around you.

As your trust in your wisdom and use it as the compass for your journey, others are inspired by you and you then are teaching by example. Others will then ask you what it is that makes you different from others and then it is time to share your journey with them.

Affirmation: "I am connecting with my inner knowledge more easily each day and I am walking the talk of my spiritual understanding."

333

You know what to do

Trust your inner knowingness. Act upon this knowledge without delay. Your angel guidance is to persist, to maintain your purpose in spite of any difficulties, obstacles, or discouragement; continue steadfastly toward your desired goal. Often times one gives up on their dreams right before they are seeing the manifested results of all the hard work they have done.

Remember to hold the visions of your desires. If this is a vision of what someone else wants for you or have you do, and it is not a part of your goals, and they do not bring you the satisfaction of a job well done. Chances are that when you consult your inner knowingness, desires and passion, you will choose to follow a different path.

What lies in your heart? If it isn't your passion, gently let it go with love, and move on to that which brings you joy, peacefulness, balance and harmony. When you are happy, those who love you will see the light of all that you experience, and the power this creates. This is how the world changes, 'One courageous soul at a time.'

Affirmation: "I am living in higher purpose right now. I follow my heart and I do what I love from moment to moment."

334

What are your dreams

This is a magical time, Make a wish, and be prepared to enjoy its manifestation. As you make your wish, **know** that it will indeed come true. It may not come exactly as you imagine, so hold the thought of the final outcome and the feeling that bringing it your way will bring to you. Your angel guidance is to trust in your inner wisdom and the service of your angels to bring you to your goals and to be with every step of the way, guiding and supporting you.

Ground your dreams in the physical realm. Sit quietly so that you can find the stillness within, Then you can shine a pure, clear light into every area of your life.

We are here helping you balance the spiritual and material so that you can enjoy a fulfilling Earthly adventure.

Affirmation: "I am magical and create my dreams by following my inner guidance."

335

Discipline

A little bit of self discipline goes a long way. Through discipline comes spiritual freedom. The master you are called on to obey is your Higher Self. You are an aspect of a part of you that is connecting to everything and all that is. You came to earth on a mission and together with your higher self and the perspective they offer you and self-discipline, you will fulfill it more quickly.

Be cautious of overindulgence as this time. While it seems fabulous in the moment, as you wake up, and you will wake up, you feel 'hung-over' when you are done. All temptations are there: the truly amazing people are those who can look, taste, but don't get carried away with them. If you go overboard on any aspect of your life, you may not like how you feel tomorrow. Your entire being begins to feel out of focus, balance and rhythm.

Tune in and ask your angels for their help and support so that your life becomes more happy and rewarding and divinely directed. Take some time out to recharge, reconnect and reinvigorate your batteries regularly.

Angel wisdom reminds you that you are a powerful creator. When you focus on the next dream, idea or desire, with discipline, you will create your dreams. Discipline is a key to fulfilling your destiny.

Affirmation: "Self discipline brings me freedom."

336

There are no accidents

Everyone and every situation are placed on your path for a purpose.

Your angel guidance is to ask your angels to help you find the purpose within your current path. It may be to strengthen you, or offer you an opportunity to resolve or forgive something from the past. It can be to release old patterns, or simple to bring more happiness and joy into your life.

Ultimately the purpose for most of your experiences is to bring more joy, satisfaction and fulfillment to your life, although it doesn't always feel that way when you are going through a particularly trying time. Seek the soul qualities of that which you desire. Laughter, joy, and balance will help to place you on the path to your destiny.

You are also reminded to keep at it, for it may be that new doors are opening for you as you find the gift within each experience. Gratitude for the past and present are keys to creating in your future and your now.

Affirmation: "I am ready for all the opportunities before me."

337

The power of joy

Everything is how it needs to be right now.

Look past the illusion of how you think things should be and see the underlying order around you. Regardless of where you find yourself, you always have the choice to feel joy. Joy carries a very high vibration that can heal and transform any situation or relationship.

Your angel guidance is to visualize any situation that you feel is 'less than' being infused with love and feelings of joy that you once felt when you began that particular journey. See the lessons and the love that it has taught you and release everything else. Be patient with yourself and others and trust in the higher forces to know what the next best step is for you take at this time. Your angels can see all the angles that perhaps you cannot, therefore, ask your angels to enfold you in their beautiful wings and listen to the promptings of the Divine and they share with you.

Affirmation: "All Things happen in the most perfect way at exactly the right time."

338

Healing hearts

Let the angels open your heart, for it is now time to heal old wounds. Ask us for help with any aspects of relationships that need healing. Know that all relationships ultimately have blessings, growth lessons, and love at their core, even if appearances seem otherwise. Stay focused upon truth as much as possible. Ask us to help you see the other person's point of view, or all sides to any unhealed situations.

Trust that the Universe has an infinite supply of love available to everyone and that each one will find the path that is right for them and just love them, love them regardless of all outside appearances. Lean on us for strength and courage, and take good care of yourself. Visualize everyone involved (including yourself) surrounded in soft pink lights, being cooperative, open minded, and compassionate. Trust the inner guidance that you receive and know that changes are sometimes uncomfortable; however they are a part of evolution and growth and a wonderful sign from the Universe.

Affirmation: "My heart is open and healing. I trust in the goodness of the Universe."

339

Take a spiritually based re'treat'

You are the most important person in your life, take a respite and spend some time with yourself, and your angels. Get to really know your true self with all of your amazing dreams, goals and projects.

Take some time and ease back from all the drama that is surrounding you. Snuggle on the sofa with an enlightening book and relax. This is an opportunity to take a mental health break from the world around you.

There has been a lot of shifts happening in the heart and finances for many, and a new period of stability is coming that will allow you the opportunity to find your footing through all these changes. Spend some time recouping and recovering, and taking care of you. Ask your guardian angels to commune with you during your time out and spend some time in dialogue with them.

The guardian angels say, *"We are here always to support you so that you can grow spiritually, you are never alone and we are always with you. So take a time out and spend some time with us, and you will feel stronger and clearer as you move forward."*

Affirmation: "I take time and space for myself to evolve and expand my light."

340

Steady progress

You are making progress, even if you can't see what is coming up next, trust that you are exactly where you should be at this time to learn and understand and evolve as the beautiful light that you are. Keep marching forward with your chin up and if you have clearly stated what path you wish to take, follow the path that seems the brightest. Keep your dreams in your heart and find the joy where you are at as you move forward. It does not have to be fast, for this is not a race and slowing down to enjoy the scenery along the way. Let your guides and your angels take care of the details of how your miracles unfold, just expect them, look for them, and they are there.

Enjoy and celebrate each step along the path. There is always a choice and you can always choose joy regardless of the circumstances. Smile, let the love of your angels flow out of your heart and engulf all of you in the wave as it pours slowly around you, enveloping you, cocooning you and stay in the moment. Then when you are ready, open your eyes and continue on. Change is always going to happen, as that signifies evolution, and that is what you came here to experience.

Affirmation: "I am engaged in activities everyday that help me make my dreams a reality."

341

Honour

Honour yourself and follow your guidance. Many of you have been undergoing tremendous spiritual growth. With all the shifts and changes that have been happening to you, you begin to honour yourself more and trust your inner guidance. The more you use and trust your inner wisdom, the more it grows. Whatever you feed shall grow exponentially, and we see so much happening on your earth plane by those of you who are becoming so bright.

Take some time today to go out and play. Being out of doors and having some fun will assist in your shifts. You are able to breathe fresh air and expand your lungs as you run about laughing and enjoying yourself and from this, fresh new ideas pop into your head from your entourage of Light Beings, as well as your higher self. Drink plenty of life giving water too.

As you find more joy on journey each day becomes brighter than the one before it.

Affirmation: "I connect and trust my inner wisdom. I am vibrating at higher levels each day. I honour and love myself."

342

Light

Light illuminates the dark and brings with it hope and inspiration. Ask your angels to fill you with more light any time you feel you want to raise your vibration. As your light becomes stronger and clearer, you will find more clarity and purpose. As you radiate brightly and become a beacon, you gain confidence that assists you in moving forward towards your dreams.

Ask your angels to light your path, to increase your spiritual connection so you better trust what is the next best step to take and trust that all is enfolding before you in a most magnificent way. Expect miracles and they will occur.

Trust that you dearly loved and supported. Lean upon us if your confidence waivers and we will buoy your courage and faith.

Affirmation: "I am increasing my ability to experience and express more love each day."

343

Blossoming

You are just getting started. Have patience with yourself and the process, and do not give up. Angel wisdom reminds you that sometimes the process takes longer than expected so be gentle with yourself. Open up to compassion, but most of all access the wisdom within that recognizes the Divine in everyone and everything including and especially yourself.

Know that you, your loved ones, and your possessions are safe and protected by the angels. Trust in yourself and the beauty that is you and know that when you are true to yourself you spread much light, joy and freedom and empower others to find the good in themselves as you share the beauty of who you are.

Affirmation: "I am focused, expanding and empowered more and more each day."

344

Flow of prosperity

Let the flow of prosperity open up for you. You now have the opportunity to connect with the flow of universal abundance, to transform all of your thoughts and desires into tangible form. Tap into your manifesting power by focusing on abundance instead of worrying about having enough money, love or time. The angels wish to remind you that you have nothing to fear. A new flow of prosperity is supporting you now and your prayers have been heard and answered.

Love yourself enough to set boundaries with others and say no to demands on your energy and time that does not match your agenda and use all of that energy to focus on that which you desire. Release projects and people and thoughts that are not focused energy on your desired path.

Affirmation: "I will allow the abundant good of the Universe to manifest through me now; in my mind, body, emotions and activities."

345

Meditate daily

Daily meditations will change your life. Meditation offers you so many opportunities to take charge of your journey. It helps to bring you clarity; it will improve your health. It connects you to your guides and your angels and is a wonderful way to nurture yourself. WE cannot emphasis enough, the assistance that a regular meditation practice will bring into your life.

Connect with the still, quiet place within your heart, for we are always there waiting to talk with you. And from this space of connection your heart opens and expands, allowing you to be more in love with your earth journey. Use affirmations daily to assist in keeping you in that space of love. Affirmations can open the floodgates to your ability to manifest that which you desire and also assist in keeping your focus and clarity along the way.

Affirmation: "I radiate love, light, harmony and compassion from my heart center."

346

Friendship

Changes in your friendships are occurring.

Be lovingly honest with yourself and your friends at this time, and enjoy the benefits of a true friendship.

As you change on the inside, your life begins to change on the outside. Amongst these are changes in your relationships with family and friends.

Changes in friendship are natural. As you begin to vibrate at a different rate you will attract new, healthier friends and relationships to you. Let go and surrender your relationships to the angels. Know that we are with you supporting these natural changes to match the new you. Never fear you will be alone, for we are always with you and you are never ever alone.

You are ready for the next step in your relationships and new friendships with people who better mirror your interests and ambitions.

Affirmation: "I support the success and happiness of everyone I know and they support my success and happiness as well."

347

Movement

Feeling stuck or indecisive? Now is the time to tune into your intuition.

Trust your feelings, let go of self doubt, even in the face of others opinions. Your spiritual sensitivity helps you see the truth. Although it may be easier to go with the crowd, or to shrink into apathy, you're called upon to take decisive action. Even if people aren't supporting you, know that spirit and the angels are. Ignore critics, or sceptics. Avoid situations or relationships that don't feel right to you.

Angel wisdom reminds you that only you know what the next best step is for you take. Focus on the stream that feeds you everything you need. Put your entire focus upon the feelings that come from tuning into your heart space and move forward from there. You desire a lifestyle that better fits the new you that is emerging. Keep your focus upon what you truly desire.

Let go of that which no longer serves you and move forward in creating that which desire, you are ready to move forward now!

Affirmation: "Each step I take brings me closer to my purpose and desires."

348

Explore your options

It is time to look at other possibilities.

It is a good time to make changes and look at all the options and possibilities that are before you now, for there is always more than one path that leads you where you want to go. Ask an expert or someone that you respect to assist you in seeing the bigger picture if it feels like your options are not there, for there are always choices to me made.

Focusing on service, or "How may I serve" is also a way to open up the stream of giving and receiving, which opens up the streams of new thought. Find a project that feeds your soul and allows you to serve in a way that brings you joy as this puts you in a stream of bliss. This stream can feed you everything you need and help to open doors that may have been previously closed or open new ones that you never thought would be open to you.

Affirmation: "I am open to all possibilities. I see all the blessings and gifts in my life."

349

Trust your Divine guidance

You are indeed hearing us. You are being helped; we are working behind the scenes to assist in making things happen, even if you haven't seen the results yet, trust and don't give up now. Your desires are coming to fruition. Keep up the good work and trust and believe that all things are possible for you.

Trust the divine guidance that you feel within your heart. Trust your heart. We are always with you guiding you with thoughts, words and deeds, sometimes through other human angels that are before you. Ask us to be your project assistants and then pay attention for the signs.

Affirmation: "I am empowered and enlightened through my own inner guidance and validation."

350

Be powerful

It is safe to be powerful. You know how to be powerful in a loving way that benefits others as well as yourself.

You are a powerful and strong Lightworker. The angels wish to remind you that it is time to accept and reveal your powerful self with others. Power comes from love, as your heart chakra opens you become more powerful and balanced than you ever have before. Do not be afraid. Do not fear that others may disapprove or leave you if you allow your true power to shine.

Ask your angels to assist you if your trust wavers for we are here to help you reveal your power to yourself and others in a way that enhances your relationships, self-esteem, and current life purpose. We are always by your side to lend you strength and courage; we are always by your side. Quiet your mind and open your heart and feel our love for you.

Affirmation: "I trust the Universe. I know the world is safe and working with me."

351

Trust the messages that you hear

Allow the wisdom in your heart to radiate out.

Your angels are waiting to help you in your tasks. They are

waiting to lead you toward the desires of your heart and the answers to your prayers. Please listen to and follow the steps the angels are communicating to you through your intuition, thoughts, dreams and those around you.

Meditate with us; ask to be shown your next step or answers in a way in which you understand in your current vibration if you feel you do not understand. We are always here and await your requests. Angel wisdom reminds you the prayer is the asking, and meditation is the answering. And we cannot assist without you first requesting our help.

Notice repetitious thoughts and feelings, or vivid visions, dreams or auditory messages. These are our loving messages, urging you to take action or make changes. Together we will work to co-create your answered prayers.

Affirmation: "I trust and act upon my inner guidance."

352

Unconditional love

Love yourself, others, and every situation, no matter what the outward appearance may be.

To help to heal any situation or relationship, see the other person's point of view with compassion. Instead of seeing someone or something as 'good' or 'bad', have compassion, and know that everyone is doing the best they can at the time. Instead of pitying someone, see that person's inner strength and Godliness. This encourages the Divine light to be expressed within the other person as well as yourself.

There is a solution to every problem, so look at all things with eyes of love. Focus your thoughts on the beautiful things that you can find in people or situations and raise your light above all appearances and see only love in all things.

Affirmation: "I am one with the Divine, just as you are, and it is here that I choose to reside."

353

Let your light shine

You are a Lightworker. Are you ready to shine your Divine light and love ~ like an angel ~ upon the earth and all of its beings? There are so many of you on the planet at this time for you are so dearly needed to shine your light where others dare not go.

You are sensitive to others' emotions, and it is important for you to clear yourself regularly, especially after helping someone. You can call upon Archangel Michael or your other guardian angels, to clear you of any excess energy, toxins or cords that may have resulted from your helpful efforts. You are an earth angel, and we are happy to assist you in all ways. Just Ask and we are there to assist you as you assist others.

Now is the perfect moment to embark upon service to those around you, as well as all the kingdoms of earth. So, embrace the gift that is you and share them with the world.

Affirmation: "I expand my light and I am a beacon of love and hope for those whose lives I touch."

354

Positivity

Keep your thoughts positive.

When you think and then act in positive ways, you direct a clear stream of vibrating energy directed and attracted that which you are thinking about. Use your thoughts, your words and of course your deeds in positive ways. Surround yourself with things that you love and bring you joy. This includes the humans you share your time with, what is playing on the TV or radio as this affects you too, even if you think you are not listening. Your cells are and your energy feels the vibration that is around you.

We hear you ask us for help, and sometimes you put such human stipulations on your requests that it takes longer to set everything in motion. And we here you say, "I was positive last time and look what happened, I failed." and we say, look at the vibration of what you are feeling. We see you doing your best to keep things positive and sometimes it just falls apart anyway and we say, yes, perhaps that needs to fall away too and the fastest, best way for to get there from our vantage point is to completely surrender and let go and shed all of it and then start a new, with fresh eyes and heart. It is so important to completely let it go, smile, feel our love and take the next step.

Affirmation: "I am positive and strong."

355

Perfect timing

NOW is the perfect moment to act on your inspirations.

Doors that were previously closed now are open and it is the perfect time to focus on your manifestations. It is time to be open about and honest about who and what you do. It is the perfect time to try different ventures and experiences, as this is how you grow and learn, and develop your spiritual senses.

Let the light that grows within you shine forth for others to see. It is safe to be sharing your spiritual nature with others and that light acts as a beacon to those who feel lost or alone.

Angel wisdom reminds you that you are evolving each day as you set your focused intent on those things you want to create in the physical plane. Visualize clearly using all your senses what you want to manifest and hold that vision as clearly and focused and in as much detail as possible, as if you already own it, it is yours. Ask us for assistance when you feel other thoughts that might block your manifestations and we will sweep them away. Ask us to remove any lower energy from your surroundings, the physical, emotional and mental realms, for now is the time to move forward and awaken fully to your spiritual gifts

Affirmation: "I am powerful and in control of my destiny. I trust in the Universe."

356

Supported

You are supported. You are always surrounded by an entourage of angels and guides who are ready, willing, and able to help you with all of your hearts desires. We hear you ask for help in the dark of the night and we bring you refuge, love and support, always, even when you unaware that we surround you.

Open your heart and mind to feel us, we are here. Angel wisdom reminds you that answers don't always come in the way they are expected, so open your eyes to the possibilities that are available to you now. Pay attention to the synchronicities, signs, and words that you hear. Be open to receive from others, and just be your natural loving self.

Affirmation: "I am surrounded by love and support always."

357

Work your magic

Decide clearly what you will and won't accept, as this clarity will bring immediate results. Have steady faith in a positive outcome.

You have the power to resolve any situation. Tap into your magical abilities, which you've used successfully in the past. Pull these abilities out of storage and use them to work your

magic now. Your clear and focused intentions, positive
expectations, prayers, decrees, and action steps all create the
healings and manifestations you desire.

Study alchemy and manifestation principles, for these
Universal Laws will assist you in manifesting your dreams
into reality. The more you immerse yourself in your studies
and creations, the faster they manifest in your physical realm.

**Affirmation: "I am a powerful creator and in control of
my destiny."**

358

Enjoying the outcome

It is time for you to take a moment and delight in the wonder
of everyday and celebrate in it.

Take action to take care of yourself, eat foods that nourish
your physical body, as well as your spirit. Go outside and
breathe some fresh air and marvel in all of the beauty that is
around you, as this too feeds you physically, mentally,
spiritually and emotionally. Now is the time to take action and
change those parts of your life that aren't working for you. Let
the beauty that surrounds you to sweep away old energy,
thoughts and beliefs. Make way for the new to enter.

Whenever possible celebrate with others, as you create great
energy when you are filled with laughter and lightness. Angel
wisdom reminds you to celebrate and honour all things great
or small within your life, and watch the movement and joy

that it creates for you to then manifest more of what you desire. This is creative energy at its finest.

Affirmation:"I celebrate and enjoy all aspects of my life."

359

Transform your thoughts

You are safe, and there is nothing to worry about.

As you raise your vibration, and if you read messages like these, you are shifting your vibration to higher level and therefore your creation time is less than it was before. The angels guide you to choose your thoughts carefully! Just as you are capable of manifesting masterpieces, you are also able to manifest chaos and problems. The good news is that you can also undo anything that you are unhappy with.

Angel wisdom reminds you that you are part of an awesome and benevolent team of beautiful light beings, watching over you. You are not alone and you are safe, always. Talk with your angels more frequently, like your best friend over coffee. WE are here and want to be of service at all times. Ask us to join you in your quest and become a part of your life every day.

Affirmation: "I create with every thought and emotion. Thank you for helping me to keep my focus on joy and making my dreams a reality."

360

Law of Attraction

You can change or heal any situation by elevating your thoughts to a more positive level.

You attract certain people or situations because they mirror your thoughts, emotions, and beliefs. In the same way, people and situations that you once found desirable are now moving out of your life as you've shifted your energy through your spiritual path. Remember, "Like attracts like" means that everything and everyone that you draw into your life is similar to your thought patterns.

If you want to change what or who you attract, hold more positive, loving and joyful thoughts. The guides and the angels can help you with this shift. View things as neither a reward nor a punishment, you have just attracted it, which means that you can also repel or magnify it as you choose. Visualize and affirm only what you desire.

Affirmation: "I attract what I think about and desire, I therefore carefully choose each thought."

361

What do you desire

You now have the opportunity to write the script, "What do you desire?"

Now is the time to decide what you really want to manifest in your life. Use you determination to manifest results in the physical world. You need to take control, grab those reins and move forward, and be sure you are heading in the direction in which you wish to go. Protect yourself against negativity at this time as it is often easy to become distracted and/or discouraged by other peoples thoughts and desires for you. Instead, focus on your dreams and get inspired, then move determinedly toward that which you desire to create. Be a resolute and gentle warrior.

Angel wisdom reminds you that it is inspiring when you start to take real control of your life. Meditate, keep calm, and take what action you feel guided to take. Wear blinders to naysayers and sceptics. It is your life, work on changing it for just for you. If you feel you cannot change things at this moment, work on changing how you feel about it. You always have a choice.

You are dearly loved for whatever road you take, the choice is always yours, what do you truly desire to manifest in your life!

Affirmation: "I align my desires with Spirit and my Divine self."

362

Wisdom of experience

You truly are a powerful sage, now is the time to use your experience, energy and creativity to focus on what you want to create.

Angel wisdom reminds you that you are magnificently powerful when you focus consciously on what you want to create. Now is the time to resolve and restore balance in your life. With resolute focus you will 'suddenly' see terrific things are happening without seemingly much effort. This change is the result of all the hard work you have been doing to find this balance.

Remember that your thoughts always have an effect on what happens next in your lives. It is important to be conscious of where your thoughts are at all times, so these good fortunes continue and are not just a respite after the storm. Invest wisely on all levels, the mental, emotional, spiritual and physical, you have worked hard to get where you are, and it is a great feeling to know how far you've come with all that you have learned in life's lessons.

Now is a magical moment. Feel that we are here to support and assist you whenever you ask, and celebrate the bounty in your life. You have a gold mine of resources flowing within you, now is the time to hold those loving thoughts to establish a firm flow of energy and creativity.

Affirmation: "I focus on having, being and doing. I have the power, ability, knowledge and will to create anything in my life I desire."

363

Soul growth

Stay on your present path.

You may have been going through a growth spurt of late. This is a time when you release on a spiritual, mental, and emotional level and your physical body needs time to adjust. The angels remind you to drink more water at this time, as it helps to flush and release toxins and energy that your physical body no longer needs or wants. Spend time daily in meditation and if you are able, go outside and be in nature, by a lake or the ocean if possible, at the very least with Mother Nature.

Angel wisdom reminds you that these growth sessions free up energy for a windfall of ideas and inspirations, as many forms of abundance can come your way. Be in a state of gratitude, even if there are seemingly no visible signs of this yet.

Be open to the new you that emerge from these seemingly down times in your energy and use them to your advantage. This is your opportunity for growth, health and healing, becoming that powerful you. You have the power of the Universe within you! All the power of Divine love, wisdom and intelligence is within you. You have the spiritual power to see and talk to your angels, the intellectual power to tap into the universal wisdom of the One Mind. You have the emotional power of Divine love, and physical power that is truly unlimited. Allow yourself to shine with radiant love, so that you true power shines forth and into the world in miraculous ways.

Affirmation: "I am grateful for all the divine riches I have in my life."

364

Creativity

Your soul loves to express itself.

Infuse more artistry and creativity into your life. Creativity ignites passion and excitement into your life and renews your outlook.

Close your eyes and focus on your breath and then your heart and let that energy flow over you. Then, ask yourself, "How can I bring more creativity and light into my life?" As you go about your day, your angels will drop in ideas and inspirations for your added passion.

Creativity comes in many forms and each one of you is creative in many ways. Some of you are wonderful painters, writers, and dancers, others can transform a house to a home in minutes, and some of you are great at organizing events or helping people organize themselves or their life. There are many ways to be creative.

Use your creativity to create a renewed passion for your projects and your life.

Affirmation: "My creative juices are flowing. Ideas and inspiration are part of my day, every day."

365

As within, As without

This is a time of great change and growth on a personal level as well as a global level for humanity.

As within, as without, it is a matter of process. As you change, so does the world before you.

Since those of you reading this are the healers, teachers and service workers of the Light, this is an appropriate time for this message in a time of love. There will be much spiritual growth happening and what will feel like a huge awakening. This is a good thing and what so many of you have waiting for who were awakening for the past decade or two. There is a huge rush of energy and it will be a hard time for many who do not understand what is happening and the wisdom of experiences from the teachers will be greatly sought after. This is a time to step forward Teachers and Healers as well as those who will guide others to you. Discernment is paramount at this time as there are many who will be of lesser light trying to profit from these times of change. Know that they are there to be sure there are enough of you ready for each step in order to make giant leaps and we wish to assure you there are at this time.

Trust is also another area in which many will feel tested. Staying balanced and grounded regardless of what is happening around you and trusting is the most important thing, oh and perhaps a little patience.

Remember you are also stewards of the Earth and all the beings that live upon and within her. We ask that you be conscious of the Earth and the living being that she is. And remember that each being that lives upon her is somehow an important part of her too. Just as an engine does not run properly without all of its cogs and wheels, your Earth needs all of her aspects to do what she needs to do. So, love the Earth, love the animals, and love the insects. Bless and protect all parts of her as you make your lives upon her. She is what feeds you and keeps you alive. She is what supports you, so we ask that you take the best care of her you know how. Recycle, reuse and protect all living things as you do each other.

Be strong and courageous as you face the changes. As you trust that you are these things, the changes that happen at this time will feel in flow with all things. This is the time to work on loving all things unconditionally and supporting each other on whatever path each one is taking. Each of you is evolving, it is what you came here to experience, so do not resist the change, embrace it as the proof you seek in your askings. This is the perfect time to loving assert yourself. This means to be strong and yet love in all actions. Set the boundaries that work for you and let others deal with how they face what is before them. Let them know that you love and support them regardless and then let go of any resistance. This is a time when many will face opportunities of being in more love. This can often feel like the 'rug is being pulled out from under you' if you are unprepared. Be prepared by sticking to a spiritual practice that includes time for meditation and getting clear and setting your intent from that clarity. Those of you with a spiritual practice and developing your senses and your own spiritual growth will love what is happening during this time.

Those of you who have been resisting these things will not have as much fun from a human perspective. It takes very little to shift yourself from this perspective. This is where the healers, teachers and service workers of the Light will come to get to practice more of your Lightwork. And we say it is time.

This is a magical time in your evolution. This is a wonderful time of great change. Be strong, do not hold back and be ready to soar if you choose.

Affirmation: "Each day I step further into my true power and natural way of being. I am connected to all living things and know that all things are living. I am a part of a great shifting Universe and I make a difference each day in all that I do, think and feel. I am love and share that love with everyone and everything, and so it is."

Here are some comments from Sharon's readers and listeners

"You have been in my Angel thoughts since 2008 and through all the highs and lows that are second nature to the Ascension phenomenon. You were always there with your Calling all Angels Radio Show when I needed to do some fine tuning so I could hear my Cosmic Heart Beat through the distractions. I consider you one of my dearly loved Angel friends."Jayne Mason, Australia.

"The angel messages have a way of finding you with the right message at the right time. Like a trusted friend, they gently reconnect you to the wisdom you already possess." Elena C. Illinois

"I wanted to tell you how much the angels wisdom has helped me during all this year is like having a blue print to follow sometimes you feel like you fall off the horse and when reading the angels is like they are holding your hands you have the assurance that they are there sometimes there are days where you can't make it for some reason or you have a rough day when reading them wow you feel energize splendid great it's like they are telling you "hey remember me we are here for you". THANK YOU SHARON for helping us and having the angels all the way big hug love u blessings♥♥♥" Sonia R, Florida

"Thank you Sharon and the Angels; you are my guiding light each day and the first thing I read every morning. It is as if you are speaking to me directly and that you can read my thoughts and my mind." Sarah B, British Columbia

"Sharon's sharing of her work with the angels has been a great blessing in my personal life. I have learned to "put my angels to work for me and with me." I am most grateful for the time she spends each day preparing the angel messages. They always apply to what is happening for me." Reverend Beverly Cohoon, Lemurian Healing Center, Mesa, Arizona

"I have always been in awe of the accuracy of Sharon's readings. I am a true follower of her work and read her daily. I find her to be an asset to many in guiding them along life's road. I have recommended her to many and will continue to do so. Sharon is a dear friend with a heart of gold." Dr. Rev. Theresa F Koch, author of Story of a Spirit Investigator.

"Sharon Taphorn is magically connected to the Angel Energy and shares her gifts generously and lovingly with all those who participate in her various workshops, lectures, radio shows, books and websites. I have had amazing results using the techniques Sharon has outlined on how to connect with the Angels. She is a treasure worth seeking out and spending time in her presence lifts the vibration of all she touches." Kendall F. ND Australia

For more information about Sharon, her events and workshops check out

www.playingwiththeuniverse.com .

Or sponsor a workshop in your area.

314

Join Sharon each week for 'Calling All Angels' on Thursdays at

http://www.blogtalkradio.com/shiftingtimesradio

Each week Sharon shares messages of love, transformation and healing from the Angels, Masters and other Beings of Lights, including meditations to assist in these shifting times.

At 6pm pacific/9pm eastern

Sharon presents a 2 hour free program to connect spiritual family with the guides and angels. How they can assist us in working with their energy. The program includes discussions, questions, meditations and spiritual guidance. Mini Angel Sessions are offered in the last segment of the show.

http://www.blogtalkradio.com/shiftingtimesradio

Namaste

You are Beautiful!

CPSIA information can be obtained at www.ICGtesting.com
Printed in the USA
LVOW080214270312

274845LV00003B/5/P